Searching for Health Information

Searching for Health Information

The Cancer Information Service Model

Vicki S. Freimuth

Judith A. Stein

Thomas J. Kean

upp

University of Pennsylvania Press
Philadelphia

Printed in the United States of America

Library of Congress Cataloging-in-Publication Data

Freimuth, Vicki S.
Searching for health information: the Cancer Information Service model / Vicki S. Freimuth, Judith A. Stein, Thomas J. Kean.
p. cm.
Bibliography: p.
Includes index.
ISBN 0-8122-8123-3.—ISBN 0-8122-1272-X (pbk.)
1. National Cancer Institute (U.S.) Cancer Information Service. 2. Health—Information services—United States. 3. Health behavior. I. Stein, Judith A. II. Kean, Thomas J. III. Title.
[DNLM: 1. Information Services. 2. Neoplasms—prevention & control. QZ 200 F865s]
RA645.C3F73 1989
025'.0661699'400973—dc19
DNLM/DLC
for Library of Congress 88-38116
CIP

This book is dedicated to the
Cancer Information Service staff
past, present, and future

Contents

Preface

This book is written for those who have an interest in or responsibility for disseminating information to the public. Even though the book focuses on health information, specifically cancer, it also should be useful to those communicating about other subjects. Although we make extensive use of the Cancer Information Service (CIS), a national telephone information/referral service, as a model program and the source of the data we analyze, our intention was not to write a book about the CIS. Instead, we wished to present the literature on health information seeking and contribute to that literature by analyzing the largest single data base available on active health information seeking.

The evaluation data described in the book were compiled from the standardized documentation of all calls made to the CIS for four years, from 1983 through 1986. This data base has provided a unique opportunity to study almost one and one-half million active information seekers. A second evaluation data set consists of the responses of over 7500 of these callers who were mailed a follow-up survey to assess their satisfaction with their CIS inquiry and any behavioral action stimulated. Together, these two data sources allow us to study the interaction involved in this type of active information searching. We can examine the nature of the caller and his/her inquiry, how the CIS information specialist responds to the inquiry, and finally, how the caller reacts to the information acquired.

The introduction to the book describes the general context in which people search for health information. Interest in systems to manage health information has peaked because of the evolution of the information society and the growth of health consumerism. In Chapter One, we present a theoretical overview of the nature of information and the processes people use to search for it. A model of the health information acquisiton process is developed and used throughout the rest of the book to guide our discussions. This chapter also identifies the various sources of health information which may be used by the searcher. The rest of the book focuses on one of these sources, a comprehensive telephone information/referral service, and describes the way information seeking occurs using this type of service.

The second chapter identifies issues which must be examined when developing a comprehensive health communication system and presents the CIS as a model system to show how these issues might be addressed. Chapter Three describes the CIS evaluation and presents an overview of the results for the study period. Chapter Four is the first of four chapters which examine these results in detail for each of the three user groups: the general public, symptomatic people, and cancer patients and their family/friends. Each of these chapters addresses the following questions: who are the callers, what are they asking about, what cancer sites are they interested in, how did they learn about the CIS, what behavioral suggestions were given to them, how they responded to these suggestions, and their perceptions of the information source itself.

Chapter Eight focuses on stimulating use of comprehensive communication systems like the CIS. Planned and unplanned promotion activities are explained and illustrated. Chapter Nine considers the knowledge and utilization gaps that often remain even after effective promotion activities have occurred. The knowledge gap hypothesis is examined in this chapter in light of the data from the CIS evaluation.

In the final chapter, we identify some general insights from the literature reviewed and the data analyzed which should be useful to those responsible for disseminating information to the public. This chapter also describes several foreign cancer information programs some of which were modeled after the CIS and research underway in this country, to investigate some innovative uses of this type of system to motivate behavior change.

Each of the contributing authors has had significant involvement with cancer communications and the CIS. Vicki Freimuth's research on health information dissemination over the last fifteen years has concentrated on cancer communications. In 1984, she served as a reviewer for the CIS proposals submitted to the National Cancer Institute, and subsequently was asked to help disseminate the results of the CIS evaluation efforts. Judith Stein began her involvement with the CIS in 1975 when she assisted in organizing and implementing the first operational regional office of the CIS in Miami, Florida. She joined the National Cancer Institute in 1981 as Assistant Project Officer for the CIS and served as Project Officer from 1982 to 1987. She was responsible for implementing the program evaluation that led to the data set used in the book. Thomas Kean has been actively involved in the CIS program and its evaluation from its earliest days in 1975. He was the first evaluation specialist for the Texas CIS and participated in NCI's first Evaluation Task Force to establish a standardized evaluation for CIS. In 1980, he became Project

Officer of the national CIS program and led the development of the national evaluation plan from which these data presented in the book were derived.

Many more people contributed to this book and we want to acknowledge their help. Lee Gigliotti participated in early planning discussions. Dennis George competently and cheerfully programmed and processed the CIS data bases. Melissa Dean helped analyze the user surveys. Sharon Hammond contributed to the chapter on promotion of the CIS. Thomas LeMay and Holly Broyles faithfully completed library research. Larry Kessler and Ben Hankey provided valuable insight on several important analytical issues. We are especially indebted to five reviewers who provided critical feedback to us: Erwin Bettinghaus, Peter Mansell, Rebecca Cline, Paul Van Nevel, and Kate Duffy. We also would like to thank Prospect Associates, Ltd., for their logistical and moral support. Finally, we want to thank our families for supporting us during this project.

VSF
JAS
TJK

Tables

Figures

Introduction

Each year hundreds of thousands of people in the United States die of or suffer from various diseases despite existing information on ways to prevent and detect these diseases early to reduce their impact. Cancer is one of the best examples of this needless loss and suffering. The American Cancer Society (ACS) estimated that 170,000 people died in 1987 who might have been saved with earlier diagnosis and prompt treatment (American Cancer Society, 1987). Similarly, the National Cancer Institute (NCI) targeted a 50 percent reduction in cancer deaths by the year 2000 with better application of existing knowledge and technology (National Cancer Institute (NCI), 1986). Before the public can use the prevention, detection and treatment information available, they must know what should be done and how to take action. The sheer volume of scientific information being produced as well as the complexity and contradictory nature of much of this information can overwhelm consumers as they strive to take a more active role in their health care.

Information alone does not necessarily result in improved health practices, but it is an important initial step in health behavior change. This book is designed to synthesize the existing research on health information seeking and contribute to this research by analyzing the largest single source of data on health information requests from a comprehensive communication system, the Cancer Information Service (CIS). The CIS was established by the NCI in 1975 to provide accurate, timely, and understandable cancer information to the public. Information on any aspect of cancer is provided on a one-to-one basis over the telephone by information specialists. Although the CIS handles cancer information requests the design of the system is equally applicable to other topic areas. In the following sections, the evolution of the information society and the development of health consumerism are described since they serve as significant background events influencing the health information seeking process.

The Evolution of the Information Society

We are living in the midst of an information explosion. John Naisbitt wrote in *Megatrends* (1984) that we have moved from an industrialized society to an information society and now mass produce information the way we mass produce cars. Birch (1981) reported that only 5 percent of the almost 20 million new jobs created in the 1970s were in manufacturing while almost 90 percent were in information, knowledge or service. While the total labor force grew at only 18 percent between 1970 and 1978, the number of administrators and managers grew more than three times that rate—58 percent. Naisbitt (1984) described this changing workplace:

> Today's information companies have emerged as some of the nation's largest. AT&T grossed $65 billion in 1981, far surpassing the GNP of many nations. Other information companies include IBM, ITT, Xerox, RCA, all the banks and insurance companies, the broadcasters, publishers, and computer companies. Almost all of the people in these companies and industries spend their time processing information in one way or another and generating value that is purchased in domestic and global markets. (p. 14).

Each new technological advance increases the amount of information that we can potentially use. Each year humans are able to absorb a smaller percentage of the information available in the environment (Toffler, 1970). New systems are needed for efficiently storing and accessing this enormous volume of information. Uncontrolled and unorganized information is the bane of an information society or as Naisbitt (1984) said we run the risk of "drowning in information but starving for knowledge." (p. 17).

Although this need to organize and control our expanding information base is pervasive throughout society, it is especially acute in the health field. The health care industry has grown considerably in recent years until it is now the nation's leading industry. Research is rapidly producing new information which can aid in the prevention, detection, and treatment of disease. For example:

1. Between 6,000 and 7,000 scientific articles are written each day.
2. Scientific and technical information now increases 13 percent per year, which means it doubles every 5.5 years.

3. The rate will soon jump to perhaps 40 percent per year because of new, more powerful information systems and an increasing population of scientists. That means that data will double every twenty months. (Naisbitt, 1984, p. 16).

This new information is useless to the average consumer unless it is selectively filtered through appropriate gatekeepers and translated into comprehensible language. The demand for this kind of understandable health information has been amplified by such catalysts as the consumer movement, women's rights, self-care, cost containment, informed consent, national health insurance, malpractice claims, and problems of chronic disease (Eakin, Jackson, and Hannigan, 1980).

Development of Health Consumerism

Coinciding with the information revolution has been the growth of the health consumerism movement. Health consumerism changes the traditional relationship between physician and patient because the physician's ability to make unilateral decisions is challenged and patients demand a voice in reaching closure on diagnosis and working out treatment plans. Haug and Lavin (1983) described a consumerist stance in the following way:

> it focuses on purchaser's (patient's) rights and seller's (physician's) obligations, rather than on physician's rights (to direct) and patient obligations (to follow directions). . . . In a consumer relationship, the seller has no particular authority; if anything, legitimated power rests in the buyer, who can make the decision to buy or not to buy, as he or she sees fit. (p. 213).

Haug and Lavin (1983) offered several reasons for the development of consumerism in health. First, they suggested that anti-authority attitudes and behaviors have been growing in the last two decades. Some of the most dramatic examples have been the protests against the Vietnam War, the civil rights movement, and women's liberation. For women, especially, the antiauthority actions focused on health. One of the goals of the women's movement was establishing a woman's right to make decisions about her own body.

Another impetus for the development of health consumerism was the public's increasing educational attainment. During the 1960s, the median number of years of education exceeded twelve for the first time. As consumers became more educated, they also seemed to be more willing to challenge medical authority. A literature has evolved catering to these educated consumers. Books such as *Take Care of Yourself: A Consumer's Guide to Medical Care* (Vickery and Fries, 1977) and *Playing God: The New World of Medical Choices* (Scully and Scully, 1988) and magazines such as *Prevention* and *Consumer Reports* reinforce the independent consumerism perspective.

The growth of paraprofessions in the medical field has been another impetus for the health consumerism movement. Newer occupations such as physician's assistant, nurse practitioner, and nurse midwife where non-physicians provide certain types of patient care previously reserved only for physicians, clearly demonstrate that the world of medicine is not so mysterious after all.

Probably one of the most significant reasons for the consumer movement in health is the public's increased belief in self-care. The most dramatic example of this belief has occurred in prevention, rather than treatment. The challenge of public health today is no longer infectious diseases but chronic ones, such as heart disease and cancer. The emphasis is on the individual—what one can do for one's own health and well-being. A wealth of scientific research reveals that the key to a person's health can be found in several simple personal habits: reduced smoking and drinking, diet, sleep and exercise, observing speed laws, and wearing seat belts. One study found that people who practice these seven simple health habits lived, on the average, eleven years longer than those who practiced none of them (U.S. Department of Health Education and Welfare, 1979). Even though there are many health risks that are outside the control of the individual, personal lifestyle contributes significantly to well-being.

The public is responding to the need to change to healthier lifestyles. Naisbitt (1984) provided some statistical evidence:

> At least 100 million Americans, almost half the population, are now exercising in some way—up from only about one-quarter of the population in 1960.
>
> We've reduced our fat intake mightily: Butter consumption is down 28 percent—milk and cream, down 21 percent—since 1965.
>
> Smoking, long blamed for poor health, is down substantially. . . .

> The number of health food stores in the United States increased from 1,200 in 1968 to more than 9,500 in 1982. Health food sales went from $170 million in 1970 to $2 billion in 1981. (pp. 147–48).

A final reason for health consumerism is the burgeoning concern with medical ethics. Both the public and government have had to wrestle with such difficult questions as: Is it moral to stop life support systems for a youth in an irreversible coma? to refuse an infant a heart transplant because his parents are judged incapable of caring for him? to allow a severely handicapped woman to starve herself to death? As these value questions have been debated, the public realized that they were as well-equipped as the physician to answer them.

The public's quandary is apparent. They are living in an age where knowledge is being accumulated much faster than it can be consumed. Yet if members of the public accept their role as informed consumers of health care, they must have access to the latest knowledge in prevention, detection, and treatment of diseases. This book describes one way of providing that access, through a comprehensive health communication system.

1

The Search for Health Information

Little research has attempted to describe consumers' search for this health information. Most studies acknowledge that the search for information is one step in health behavior change but are more focused on the decision-making steps. Yet, preventive behaviors, detection, and treatment options about which consumers have no knowledge cannot be chosen, no matter how much better these options might be than those of which they are aware. Similarly, criteria for decision-making have no utility to the consumer, regardless of their importance, unless they are known. The first step in understanding the information acquisition process is to understand the nature of information itself.

This chapter reviews the research on consumers' search for health information. We discuss the nature of information and present a model of the health information acquisition process. The various sources of health information are identified and illustrated.

Nature of Information

The classical definition of information is a difference in matter-energy which affects uncertainty in a situation where a choice exists among a set of alternatives (Rogers and Kincaid, 1981). Generally the motivation for seeking information is assumed to be the reduction of uncertainty. Rouse and Rouse (1984) point out a serious flaw in that assumption, however: people are uncertain about a variety of things that are of no concern to them and yet they do not seek information about them. For example, most of us are uncertain of the cost of whale steaks in Alaska, but most of us are not going to seek information to reduce that uncertainty because the topic is not important to us. Rouse and Rouse (1984) suggest that we add the concept of value or salience to our understanding of information. Is the topic for which there is uncertainty important enough for us to try to reduce the uncertainty?

Dervin (1976) extends the idea of the individual's values entering into the information seeking process. She suggests that information is more accurately defined as some unknown combination of information about reality and information that is the creative product of people. According to her view, humans take external information and organize it within their own already collected internal information, and they make sense out of their world. She presents the following three-type formulation of information:

1. $Information_1$—the innate structure or pattern of reality; adaptive information; objective information; data.
2. $Information_2$—the structures imputed onto reality by people; order created; ideas.
3. $Information_3$—the procedures by which people acquire what they didn't previously know; by which people are informed or instructed.

Dervin (1976) suggests that an explanation of human information processing is not complete unless that view looks at how people create information as well as at how they collect, store, retrieve, and use information. She asserts that, although the input of others has some utility and although individuals seek external information to close gaps in their understanding, ultimately information has value only in so far as it helps the individual to make his/her own sense out of reality.

Leventhal, Safer, and Panagis's (1983) explanation of health behavior reinforces the information-as-construction idea because it suggests that health information is understood, organized, and remembered in terms of the individual's underlying beliefs. People construct a representation of their illness and a plan to cope with it. These naive or common sense models of illness appear to be based on the integration of current symptom experience with ideas from past illness episodes and information from medical practitioners, friends, relatives, and media. Comaroff and Maguire (1981) found the same phenomenon in their study of childhood leukemia. "Parents . . . typically tried to bring the stunning diagnosis of leukaemia [*sic*] into relation with perceived medical facts, the experience of others and their own biographies and world-view." (p. 119).

Model of the Health Information Acquisition Process

Most descriptions of the information acquisition process are part of broader decision-making models, e.g., Betteman (1979). Since our focus is on the information acquisition process only, we will limit our discussion accordingly, although we recognize the importance of relating information acquired to making decisions determining health behavior. Our search for models of the information acquisition process yielded only one specifically oriented to health (Lenz, 1984). Our own model of the health information acquisition process depicted in Figure 1.1 was heavily influenced by the Lenz model as well as Atkin's (1973) model of the way information is acquired from the mass media and Betteman's (1979) consumers' information processing model. Although our model emphasizes

Health Information Acquisition Model

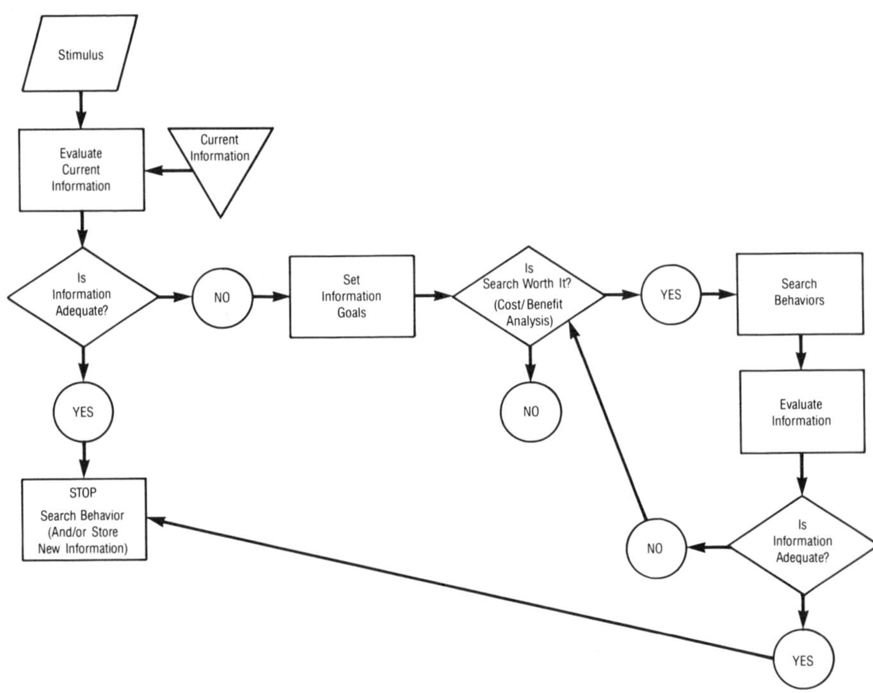

Figure 1.1

active information seeking, it also includes information acquired passively, e.g., information gained from a public service announcement (PSA) incidentally seen while watching television. In our model, this process is composed of six steps:

1. Stimulus
2. Information goals
3. Cost/benefit analysis of searching
4. Search behavior
5. Evaluation of information
6. Decision point on adequacy of information

Stimulus

The search process begins with a stimulus. Stimuli may be internal (e.g., experience of symptoms or injury) or external (e.g., PSA on television on dangers of smoking). These new stimuli are compared to the stored information from the individual's previous experience. If the individual is satisfied that his/her level of knowledge about the stimulus is adequate for decision-making, then there is no uncertainty and the information search need not be continued. A similar result occurs if a person experiences uncertainty but decides that the issue is not salient enough to warrant a further search. Suppose, for example, that the person who sees the PSA on smoking is a non-smoker. The stimulus is consistent with previous information and reinforces current behavior, so no uncertainty is created and an information search is not necessary. In many cases, however, that initial stimulus may have included new information, which is then stored to be retrieved at an appropriate time. For example, the same non-smoker may see the CIS telephone number in the PSA, store it, and later retrieve it when a friend is diagnosed as having cancer.

A more active search is stimulated in the case of the woman who discovers a breast lump, searches her memory to retrieve stored information about breast cancer, and realizes she has considerable uncertainty about its treatment and prognosis. If the topic is salient to the individual, the recognition of this discrepancy between information possessed and needed constitutes a "call to action" (Lenz, 1984) and initiates the search process.

Information Goals

Apparently people engage in information goal setting even before they actually begin the active search. They may decide in advance how soon they must have the information and what sources they will use. For example, Lenz (1979) studied community newcomers' search for information about health services and found that her subjects set time limits on their searches and decided in advance the kind of health care sources they would consult. The immediacy with which they required information was negatively related to the extent of the search. The woman who discovers a breast lump may decide that immediate action is critical and that she only trusts information coming from her physician. In such an instance her initial information search in response to the breast lump would be quite limited and immediate.

Cost/Benefit Analysis

The decision whether to engage in an active search for new information is influenced by the anticipated cost/benefit ratio. If the information search is perceived to be helpful in resolving uncertainty, then it has a high benefit value. Benefits also may include a reduction of anxiety and an increased sense of mastery or control. These benefits must be balanced against the costs involved in getting the information. Costs may include such items as delay in decision-making, financial and time expenditures, frustration, confusion, emotional distress, or decreased credibility resulting from revealing ignorance. If these costs outweigh the benefits, then it is unlikely that an active search will occur. For example, the woman who discovers a breast lump may have such an intense fear of cancer that she is not willing to incur the "cost" of seeking further information which might confirm her suspicions.

Search Behaviors

If the decision is to engage in an active search, the person moves into the key step of the process where the search behaviors are enacted. These search behaviors vary along several dimensions. The first is the *extent* of the search (usually measured as the total number of activities carried out), and includes both the *scope* (the number of alternatives investigated) and the *depth* (the number of dimensions of each alternative investigated). Most people engage in only limited information searching.

The *method* of the search refers to the information source(s) consulted. Several categories can be used to classify sources. Lenz (1984) classifies sources as impersonal (information is sought from sources such as brochures, or from a person unknown to the searcher) and personal (information is sought from an individual known personally). Betteman (1979) uses the broad classification of internal and external sources. Internal search refers to accessing information available in memory, while external refers to all sources other than memory. A better way to categorize sources is with the usual communication typology of intrapersonal (internal), interpersonal, and mass mediated (external) sources. Intrapersonal sources consist of all the knowledge, beliefs, and attitudes about health which might have been derived from earlier communication experiences. Interpersonal sources are those people who provide information, such as friends, relatives, neighbors, co-workers, or health professionals. Mass-mediated sources include print media such as newspapers, magazines, and patient education materials, broadcast media including radio, television, and telephones; and newer forms of media such as computers and videodiscs. Each of these types of sources will be described in detail following the presentation of the model.

Evaluation of Information

Information evaluation is viewed as a separate step following search behavior. After each search activity, the searcher evaluates the information gained in terms of prior information and determines once again the cost/benefit ratio. How helpful has the information been in comparison to the costs in obtaining it? Each new piece of information processed is a different health stimulus which recycles through the same process until the desired state of certainty is reached. The whole process occurs at a point in time, however, and the state of desired certainty may change with time. Immediately after diagnosis, for example, a lung cancer patient may not be able to face the facts about survival rates and may avoid that information. Two weeks later, however, this information may be necessary to achieve the desired state of certainty and the information search will persist until the information is obtained.

Decision Point on Information Adequacy

As each piece of information is acquired, the searcher must decide whether to continue the search or terminate it. This decision is a subjective one and may be influenced by the information goals set in the beginning, by a comparison between the information needed and obtained, or by a cost/benefit analysis. Betteman (1979) identifies three factors related to the difficulty of the decision which influence the amount of external search. The more easily available the information is, the more processable information is, and the less time pressure there is, the more searching will take place.

Most searches end before adequate information is found. Sometimes searches end prematurely because they seem to be yielding more frustration and confusion than insight. For example, a cancer patient may want the same questions answered by the doctor, the nurse, and printed booklets and get contradictory information from these sources. The patient is then left with the additional dilemma of assessing the relative credibility of the various sources.

Once the information acquisition is judged complete, the individual can make a decision. In addition, the new information gained during the search is stored in the memory where it can become input for future searches. A cancer patient is likely to cycle continuously through the process as new decisions confront him/her.

Sources of Health Information

Dervin and her associates (1977) describe the paradox of living in such an information-rich society that we complain of overload. Yet, studies consistently show that our citizens are uninformed about public affairs and personal concerns. Even those citizens who attempt to find information that might help often fail. This paradox exists in the health arena as well as in other areas of public affairs. A great deal of information exists but it is not very accessible to the layperson. In the following sections we will examine the major sources of this health information and highlight their strengths and weaknesses.

Intrapersonal Sources

Intrapersonal sources of health information consist of all the previous knowledge, beliefs, and attitudes about health which might have been developed from earlier communication experiences. The public's perception of cancer, for example, is frequently confused and skeptical. Rhetaugh, Anderson, and Leonard (1965) provide a vivid example of the way in which an individual's previous beliefs influence his/her perceptions.

> Mrs. Y was admitted for a diagnostic dilation and curettage. She looked so sad on the morning of her surgery that a nurse began to question her. Mrs. Y eventually opened up and expressed her feelings. She had come first into the gynecological clinic. There she was advised to come into the hospital that same evening for diagnostic surgery the following morning. She was told she could go home the day after surgery and the doctor promised to contact her with the results of the tests. The nurse discovered that the patient believed that the advice to come into the hospital on the same day that she was seen in the clinic meant that she had cancer. She was very afraid of cancer because she had had several induced abortions during her younger years. She feared that these abortions would cause cancer. She believed that cancer would be "God's way of punishing her" for her sins. The nurse contacted the surgeon who explained that the patient had been advised to come into the hospital immediately because there happened to be a bed available. He felt that she would be anxious to get back to her job and child and was surprised to hear about her strong reactions to this scheduling. When the nurse relayed the information to Mrs. Y, she was quite relieved and said, "I feel so much better. I haven't been able to talk to anyone about the things I told you in many years. I was so worried, just knew I had cancer, and I could just not imagine how my son would manage if I were to die now." (p. 22).

Obviously Mrs. Y's internalized knowledge, attitudes, and beliefs about cancer strongly influenced the way in which she processed the information from her doctor. This example reinforces Dervin's position that we create our own information.

Concrete body sensations, such as symptoms, as well as memories of past body sensations also are intrapersonal sources of health information. The importance of these body sensations is demonstrated in a study reported by Leventhal, Safer, and Panagis (1983) where 80 percent of a sample of hypertensives agreed that "people can't tell when their blood pressure is up." The frequently repeated message that hypertension has no symptoms was remembered and repeated. But nearly all of the respondents believed *they* could tell when their own pressure was elevated by such body sensations as headaches, flushed faces, and nervousness.

This study demonstrates how powerful these internalized sources of health information can be. When external information is inconsistent with our internal information, it usually is ignored.

Interpersonal Sources

The second source of health information, interpersonal communication, is important because these sources are usually trusted and hence quite influential. Not all interpersonal sources are equivalent information resources, however. Health professionals, especially doctors, usually enjoy the most credibility and influence, but are the most difficult to use because of unavailability, status differences, and tendency to use technical jargon. In a 1983 survey of the public's attitudes, beliefs, and behavior about cancer (NCI, 1983), physicians were cited as one of the most reliable and credible sources of information. However, when asked if they ever had talked to a physician about ways to reduce their chances of getting cancer, nearly 86 percent of the respondents said "no," (NCI, 1983). Many patients may have questions for their physicians but are hesitant to ask them because they are afraid to reveal their ignorance, are reluctant to take up too much of the physician's time, or are afraid to question a strong authority figure.

Waitzkin's (1985) report of 336 encounters between 34 doctors and 314 of their patients illustrates some of these difficulties in patient/physician communication. He found that in an average encounter of 16 minutes, the doctor spent 1.3 minutes or less than 9 percent of the time giving information, yet the doctors perceived that they had spent almost seven times that long providing information. Patients averaged 8 seconds asking questions, or 1 percent of the encounter. The patient asked 2.8 questions in a typical interaction and the doctor provided 7.1 explanations, 29 percent of which were in response to questions and 71 percent which were spontaneous explanations. In 28 percent of these question/answer exchanges, there were discrepancies between the technical level of the question and its answer. Waitzkin (1985) also discovered some reasons for the variation in information giving in the medical encounter. More information was given the poorer the prognosis, the longer the doctor had known the patient, the higher the socio-economic level of the patient, and the less busy the doctor.

Doctors are not the only health professionals used by patients as information sources. Nurses are often more accessible to patients and sometimes will share information even when told to withhold it (McIntosh 1974). However, nurses also use strategies to discourage information seeking. They may, for example, feign busyness in order to make themselves unavailable to answer questions. They also may view questions as complaints and communicate subtly to patients that they should not be asked (McIntosh, 1974).

Another, often overlooked, interpersonal source of information is the fellow patient. McIntosh (1974) cites evidence that tuberculosis patients and even child polio patients discuss their disease among themselves and compare themselves with other patients to judge their own condition. Self-help and volunteer patient groups, such as Reach to Recovery, Make Today Count, and I Can Cope, are proof of the need cancer patients have to communicate with each other. This need for communication with others in similiar situations may vary with stages of the illness. For example, Comaroff and Maguire (1981) found that leukemia patients and families had an intense need to identify with others who had the same affliction at times of crisis, such as initial diagnosis, relapse, and death. But when definitions of the illness had reached relative stability, and hence the search for meaning was satisfied, referencing decreased and other patients were avoided since they were possible sources of disorienting information.

Other interpersonal sources of information are those individuals seen on a regular basis but who are only superficial acquaintances (called "weak links" in the social support literature). These sources have been called community gatekeepers or urban agents, and might include teachers, bartenders, hair dressers, and grocery checkers. These superficial acquaintenances are particularly rich sources of new information.

Finally, the most familiar interpersonal sources are family and close friends. From these interpersonal sources one might compare symptoms, borrow remedies, refer one another for treatment, and comment on one another's appearance. Even though the health professionals are always rated as the most credible sources, they are not consulted as frequently as lay persons. Perhaps patients find lay persons more accessible and are more comfortable talking to them. Indeed, O'Reilly (1982) concluded that accessibility of the source consistently determines usage.

Miller (1973) studied this kind of lay consultation by interviewing 139 head and neck cancer patients about the advice they sought when they first suspected a problem. Sixty-two percent of these individuals first discussed the problem with medically uninformed sources, 26 percent consulted with medically informed persons, e.g., friends who were also health professionals, and only 12 percent went directly to a health professional. Miller (1973) concluded that this use of lay consultation did not delay patients from seeking professional care but was a positive force in encouraging them to seek appropriate care.

The public faces a dilemma in using interpersonal sources for health information. Those persons who have the most authoritative information are the least accessible to them. Consequently, the less authoritative but more approachable interpersonal sources are more likely to be used.

Mass Media Sources

The third type of informational resource is mass media. Mass media may disseminate health information both deliberately through campaigns designed specifically to have this impact and incidentally through entertainment programming that contains health-related information. When asked directly in surveys, the public credit the mass media as the source of most of their health information. In 1978, the American Cancer Society (Lieberman, 1979) found that the most often mentioned source of cancer information was mass media. Eighty-two percent of the sample reported that they heard about cancer on television, 65 percent through newspapers, 61 percent through magazines, and 42 percent through radio. The 1983 NCI survey asked about sources of *cancer prevention* information and found that the most frequently reported sources of information were magazines (64%), newspapers (60%), and television (58%). There are several limitations to these survey-based analyses of health information sources. First, people usually are asked to recall sources of information used in the past. We are then relying on people's self-perceptions of their information, or where they think they get health information. Even if they could recall accurately, we are not measuring influence of the information or whether the information prompted any health actions. Robinson and Levy (1986) also tried to determine the primary information source for knowledge of current events. They exploded the myth that television is the main source of the public's news. In fact, they denigrate the whole approach of trying to determine the most important source of information, arguing that the public employs a variety of information sources.

Studies of mass media effects over the last several decades have moved from simplistic descriptions of a "hypodermic needle" effect, a direct and universal response to the media, to a two-step flow model, where messages flow from the media to opinion leaders who then disseminate them to others, to more recently, a multi-step flow model, where messages can reach audiences directly and/or through many layers of interpersonal contacts (Rogers, 1983).

Relationship Between Mass Media and Interpersonal Communication

There is considerable agreement that the primary function of the mass media is to create awareness and reinforce existing behavior, whereas interpersonal sources can influence change. Chaffee's (1972) reference to the "interpersonal context of mass communication" perhaps best describes the complex, transactional interplay of media and interpersonal sources in the diffusion of information. He strengthens the case for a dynamic exchange among senders and receivers by citing evidence that individuals' choices of media are often related to their social contacts and that individuals' use of media can be motivated by "communicatory utility;" i.e., individuals selectively retain information they believe to be congruent with the views of those with whom they expect to communicate at some future time. Butler and Paisley (1977) describe this complex network in the following way:

> From the time the information is born as a concept within the communication program to the time it modifies a person's image in such a way as to produce desired outcomes, the message may have traveled over several networks and through many phases of transformation, some of them external to the person, others internal. (p. 9).

Slaughter, Napolitano, and Freimuth (1985) studied information sources used by mothers deciding whether to get their infants immunized with DPT. They found support for the transactional interplay of media and interpersonal sources. Mass media represented a majority of first sources of the DPT controversy but quickly declined as a source for subsequent communication, thus reinforcing mass media's role as a vehicle for creating awareness and stimulating public discussion. Further support on mothers' decisions to vaccinate their children with DPT was only moderate (an average of 3.7 out of a possible 7 on a scale measuring strength of influence); the primary effect of mass mediated sources was to raise uncertainty rather than to strengthen existing beliefs about the vaccine. Conversely, health professionals and other interpersonal sources occurred less frequently as first sources but increased in frequency as subsequent sources.

Robinson and Levy (1986) summarize this relationship between mass and interpersonal communication is the following way:

> To a large extent information does not sink in (or become "deep processed") until it has been tested and evaluated against the norms and attitudes of one's peers and colleagues. (p. 234.)

Problems in Mass Mediated Coverage of Health

Sandman (1976) suggests the mass media can influence the health consumer in a number of ways:

1. Need manipulation through direct advertising appeals.
2. Salience manipulation where there is an attempt to increase or decrease the importance of an existing attitude or belief.
3. Reinforcement of already developed habits and tendencies.
4. Legitimization of current practices and practitioners.
5. Establishment of the public agenda regarding critical medical problems worthy of national attention.
6. Provision of models of health behavior to be imitated.

However, there are several problems inherent in the types of health information the mass media can provide. First, tensions exist among scientists, science reporters, and editors as to what is appropriate health information to cover. Because the mass media deal in fragments of air time and print space, information must be tightly packaged by writers and editors which often results in oversimplification. Scientific research is a slow process in which knowledge is built incrementally. Yet media like to cover sensational, fast-breaking events.

Journalists who cover the scientific news frequently are referred to as an "inner club" (Dunwoody, 1980), a mutually reinforcing community of professionals who rely on each other and share information, the result of which is homogeneity of content and avoidance of conflict in science reporting.

Mass media also are vulnerable to pressures from advertisers on whose revenue they depend. Many researchers claim mass media's coverage of the dangers of smoking has been limited because of the fear of alienating large cigarette advertisers. Whelan, Sheridan, Meister, and Mosher (1981) completed a study of 12 years of women's magazine coverage of the health hazards of tobacco. Of 548 articles and columns about health topics in 12 magazines, only 12 articles were classified as anti-smoking.

Finally, many health issues, such as cancer, are emotional issues and subject to highly personalized interpretations. For example, a news article about an experimental treatment might raise unrealistic hopes in a cancer patient regardless of how carefully the writer qualified the expectations for the treatment.

Types of Media

Newspapers

Studies of newspaper coverage of cancer in 1977, 1980, and 1984 (Greenberg, 1986) provide evidence of some of these problems. In general, the newspaper coverage in all three years did not include much helpful information for people trying to minimize their chances of getting cancer. The majority (73%) of news content about cancer was hard news of timely events. Feature stories ranged from 7 percent in 1977 and 1980 to 11 percent in 1984. Seven percent of the clippings in 1984 were health columns and only 3 percent were in-depth articles. Cancer topics which might be helpful to consumers, such as prevention, coping, and survival rates, received minimal coverage compared to the focus on cancer causation. Cancer causation and treatment were the most frequent topics of cancer news in 1984, accounting for 57 percent of all articles. Environmental carcinogens, particularly the pesticide EDB, received three times more coverage than lifestyle causes of cancer.

The little coverage that did exist on cancer prevention/risk reduction centered on measures government agencies could take rather than on what individuals could do to reduce risk. Only 12 percent of the 1984 stories analyzed covered NCI's cancer prevention campaign messages which emphasized what people could do to minimize their own cancer risk.

Coverage of cancer as a disease was general, without reference to specific body site, which further contributed to the misconception of cancer as a singular disease rather than over 100 different diseases with different symptoms, treatments, and prognoses.

Moreover, cancer patients could not turn to newspapers for information on coping with the disease. The articles emphasized dying rather than coping. Less than 5 percent of any of the stories mentioned resources for coping. Even the health columns analyzed included very little information on coping with cancer and resources available. Thus, very little direct emotional support or even information on where to find emotional support was available through the newspapers.

Magazines

Magazines have some advantages over newspapers as health information sources. First, most newspapers must appeal to broad general audiences. Magazines, however, often have quite narrow audiences and can more easily be targeted to a group interested in health issues. Naisbitt (1984) reports that there are over 13,000 special interest magazines. Several of these are specifically focused on health (e.g. *Prevention* and *American Health*). Many other magazines appeal to fitness enthusiasts (e.g., *Shape* and *Runners' World*) or dieters (e.g., *Weight Watchers*). Moreover, most women's magazines, whether appealing to the homemaker (e.g., *Good Housekeeping* and *Better Homes and Gardens*), the career woman (e.g., *Working Woman* and *Self*), or the young single woman (e.g., *Cosmopolitan*), recognize women's interest in health and carry health features regularly. In fact, a new magazine introduced in 1986 is targeted just at cancer patients. *Cope* is the first non-medical publication ever to be written for the cancer family. It is not designed to give medical advice or clinical information on treatment. Instead it promises to bring "news of ideas to enhance capacity to cope successfully with cancer and master the lifestyle changes imposed by the illness." Merrill G. Hastings, Jr., the publisher, started this magazine when his wife became a cancer patient and he became personally aware of the importance of information as an "antidote for fear."

Second, magazine articles frequently can devote proportionately more space to a health issue than can newspapers. Newspapers have more demands on their space and less lead time to develop in-depth analyses.

Patient Education Materials

Some of these limitations of the news media coverage of health are overcome in the specialized media information sources known as patient education materials. These materials usually consist of pamphlets, booklets, and audio-visual programs which can be targeted more specifically and can present more detailed information about the health problem. The following are examples of some of the patient education materials available:

> "Taking Time—Support for People with Cancer and the People Who Care about Them" is a booklet for persons with cancer and their families, addressing the feelings and concerns of others in similar situations and how they have learned to cope.
>
> A cassette tape and booklet for adolescents with cancer which focuses on the special concerns of the adolescent including relationships with parents, peers, and health professionals, school attendance, and body image.

"Financial Aspects of Coping with Cancer—A Primer for the Patient and Family" is a booklet which addresses financially related aspects of the disease.

Even those materials, however, must present information which will meet the typical patient's needs and cannot respond uniquely to each patient. We know that patients need different kinds of information depending on timing, whether they have just been diagnosed or are recovering. Yet Evans and Clarke (1983) report that most information on cancer given to patients is cognitive in nature and is given within 24 to 48 hours after diagnosis. Patients also are more receptive to different sources at different points in the treatment process. At some points, a physician may be the best source, at others, a successful former patient, someone in the same stage of treatment, or a significant other. Different health care situations, e.g., certainty of treatment outcome, length of regimen, and unpleasantness of side effects of treatment should also be considered in preparing these materials.

Health professionals often fail to acknowledge the importance of these educational materials to patients. Messerli, Garamende, and Ramano (1980) found that nearly 80 percent of surgeons surveyed provided no written information to patients, although breast cancer patients indicated that printed materials were very important sources of information.

Television—Public Service Announcements

Several forms of broadcast media are used for health information. We are familiar with public service announcements (PSAs) on both radio and television. "Fight cancer with a check-up and a check" and "Do it for the loved ones in your life" are two well-known slogans from PSAs. PSAs, however, have some serious limitations. Because the air time is donated, not purchased, PSAs often are aired in the hours when the number of viewers is quite low. Moreover, PSAs must be very brief messages, usually no more than 30 seconds. And PSAs have to compete with slickly produced commercial advertisements both for air time and for audience attention. According to Mendelsohn (1976) each of us encounters some 350 mass communicated commercial messages daily, plus countless public service messages.

Campaign planners are often naively optimistic about the potential reach of their PSAs. From their distribution to gatekeepers, these PSAs progress through a narrow funnel-like process where the gatekeeper controls the messages' potential exposure. Hammond, Freimuth, and Morrison (1987) tracked the PSAs which were used in the NCI's Cancer Prevention Awareness Campaign through this funnel process. Based on Nielsen figures for October 1985 of the U.S. population over 18 years old with television sets, it was estimated that the potential audience for the campaign was over 170 million. An analysis of Broadcast Advertiser's Reports (BAR) for the NCI campaign showed that the PSAs were aired 5030 times during a 21 month period. During this time, BAR estimates that 28.18 percent of the total television homes were exposed to the messages. Using the Nielsen population figures and assuming two adults per household, this percent of exposure equals 24 million people having potentially viewed the PSAs, only 14 percent of the original target group. The impact of television PSAs will be discussed more fully in Chapter Seven.

Television—Health Programs

There are only a few regular health programs on television and several programs such as "Sixty Minutes," the network morning news shows, and women's shows which regularly discuss health topics. Dr. Art Ulene created the Cable Health Network in 1982 as an ambitious attempt to provide programming dedicated primarily to health concerns. The attempt failed because of low ratings and low advertising revenues. Cable Health Network was merged with another cable service, Daytime Network, to become the new Lifetime and has evolved to become more entertainment than health education. Occasionally, there are special programs devoted to health issues, such as a 3-hour NBC documentary on health care in America in 1978, a 1981 nationally televised "heart test" conducted for audience participation in ABC's "20/20" program, and the extensive exposure given to AIDS in the last few years. Some of the programs are more likely to be aired on PBS than on commercial television. One of these early PBS specials was "Joan Robinson: One Woman's Story," a documentary of a middle-aged woman from Massachusetts who was dying from cancer. Through this program, Robinson allowed the audience an intimate look at the physical and emotional trauma she faced. Another PBS special, "Why Me?" featured eight women who had surgery for breast cancer and openly discussed their personal experiences. Nationwide surveys discovered that the majority of women who had viewed the program had favorable responses and found it helpful. One woman summed it up, "Now I know what breast cancer is all about, and I think I could handle it if it struck me personally." Health programs on television can provide significant information to the public if they are able to attract the public's attention to watch.

Television—Entertainment Programs

Since the single largest nonsleeping activity outside the workplace is watching television (McDonald, 1986), this medium has the potential of communicating considerable health information incidentally in the plots of entertainment programs. Long (1978) reported a study which asked respondents about health information learned from dramatic shows and found that 48 percent of those who watched them reported getting some useful information from them.

Yet there are real concerns about the accuracy of this "useful" information. A study (Turow and Coe, 1985) in which the treatment of illness on all three networks was examined over a two week period (90.5 hours), revealed 723 interactions in which ill people appeared. Most of these ill people appeared in either commercials or entertainment programs. Even though cancer is responsible for more deaths each year than any other disease except heart disease, only 1 percent of the ill people depicted had cancer. Turow and Coe (1985) only examined portrayals of illness. Gerbner and his associates (1981) analyzed health-related content of more than 1600 programs over a ten-year period. They concluded:

> Prime-time characters are not only healthy (though often vulnerable to inflicted injury) but despite all the mayhem, eating, and drinking, are also relatively sober, safe from accidents, and slim at all ages. They hardly ever need glasses (even in old age, only one in four wears them) and rarely suffer impairment of any function.
>
> Obesity, a problem that plagues from 25 to 45 percent of this country's population . . . claims few victims on television. . . .
>
> Despite all the violence on television, the leading causes of violent injury and death—industrial and highway accidents—are rare. Moreover, television characters rarely take precautions against them. (p. 903).

Sometimes health issues are handled accurately and sensitively such as the two-part episode about breast cancer on "Cagney and Lacey," a popular series about two policewomen. However, when Smith, Trivax, Zuehlke, Lowinger, and Nghiem (1972) monitored a typical 130 hour broadcast week of a commercial network television channel in Detroit, they found that health-related content appeared only 7.2 percent of the time; furthermore, that 70 percent of this health material was inaccurate or misleading or both. Unfortunately no update of this study has been completed, so it is not possible to assess the accuracy of current health portrayals. We do know from Turow and Coe's (1985) study that few models of effective coping behavior were available in recent television programs. Of 723 illness episodes analyzed, only 10 percent involved coping. Only two of the 248 commercials referred to coping and only 18 percent of the noncommercial illness episodes depicted psychological aspects of coping with the problem. One of the few models of coping available in the televised illness episodes was that of a heart patient who listened to classical music to keep her mind off her upcoming transplant.

One of the most controversial medical entertainment programs was "St. Elsewhere," a weekly, hour-long drama that attracted an estimated 18 million people. Some of the show's major themes included the fallibility of doctors, strained relations among staff or between doctors and patients, the daily mingling of humor and tragedy, and the ethical dilemmas inherent in the practice of medicine. A medical show such as "St. Elsewhere" is likely to have its own medical advisor; for a show that only occasionally covers medical issues the Hospital Advisory Council and the Physicians Advisory Committee on Radio, TV, and Motion Pictures help writers and producers keep the information and scenes presented factual and accurate.

Patients may react to these programs differently than the general public. One former fan of "St. Elsewhere" had been unable to watch since she had lung surgery. She said her hospital experience "was amazingly similar. It was the pitch, the fever pitch. . . . It's recreating something I really choose to forget." (Okie, 1986).

These entertainment programs can be powerful sources of health information for their viewers. Fictional characters can become models of how to prevent, detect, treat and cope with illness. Fictional doctors can create expectations of physician behavior that are difficult for real doctors to live up to. Sandman (1976) offers a list of beliefs about medical practice that are likely to be generated or reinforced by viewing health-related content on television:

1. That doctors are kind, generous, handsome (male, of course), fearless, and heroic, while sensitive to the personal and psychological needs of their patients (female, of course).

2. That the best, indeed often the only, solution to a host of medical problems is surgery.

3. That access to medical care is quick, non-discriminatory, and apparently costless, since television doctors treat one patient at a time, and never discuss fees.

> 4. That if anyone is at fault in the health production process, it is the patient who characteristically hides vital, perhaps embarrassing, information from the doctor, who has to tease it out finally at the end of a dramatic, tearful confrontation.
>
> 5. In those rare instances where radical, experimental surgery or chemotherapy is not the solution to medical problems, the victim is still to be blamed, as the problem is discovered to lie in some psychological problems uncovered by the physician-detective. (p. 581, n 9).

Radio

Much less is known about the use of radio as a health information source. When asked on surveys, people generally do not credit radio as an important source of health information. Schwartz has a different interpretation of what he calls the "most invisible and emotional of all media." (Media's Muscleman, p. 64).

> People don't remember radio as a source of information because they don't consciously listen to it. Rather, they bathe in it and sit in it. Just as we are not conscious of breathing, we are not actively aware of radio-mediated sound in our environment. Yet we are deeply involved with radio, and we are strongly affected by radio programming that allows us to participate. (Media's Muscleman, p. 65).

Even though people do not consciously credit radio as a source of health information, this medium could be responsible for much of the more passive information acquisition.

The coverage of health on radio is similar to that of television except that radio has far more talk or interview programs where a guest expert may discuss a health topic and listeners can call in and ask questions of that expert. Little research has been done on use of this format for information seeking.

Telephone

The source of health information we will focus on in this book is the telephone, an interesting cross between a mass medium and an interpersonal source. Altman (1984) suggests that the "advantage of health telephone programs is that they combine some of the positive components of mass media—high exposure, convenience, cost-effectiveness, user anonymity—with some of the positive components of face-to-face interactions—personalized attention." (p. 21). A CIS caller expressed the advantages of the telephone quite well when she said: "I cannot discuss personal matters with friends and relatives; I can with strangers, on the phone." (Altman, 1984, p. 319). Cherry (1977) argues that the telephone has a more profound social effect than other media because it continues the verbal tradition: it operates with the human voice and requires no special codes, training, or skills. She emphasizes the psychological value of the telephone:

> Every time we hold a conversation we relate to another person, not to a thing; their replies to our remarks reinforce the sense of our existence. We are challenged and valued—our partner is a mirror in which we see our own images. We exist as persons, through society. (p. 123).

Because the telephone eliminates the visual channel present in a face-to-face encounter, researchers have been interested in the relative effectiveness of the two means of communication. In two field experiments, Catanzaro and Green (1970) compared three methods of communication, face-to-face, telephone, and letters, and found that they did not differ in persuasive impact, except that commitments made face-to-face were more likely to be followed by compliance than commitments made on the telephone. Janofsky (1971) also compared these sources but was interested in a different criterion variable, willingness to self-disclose. In a ten minute experimental interview between strangers, interviewees were equally willing to talk about themselves and express their feelings on the telephone and in face-to-face interviews. Reid (1977) concluded from his study comparing face-to-face communication with telephone communication:

> In information transmission and problem solving conversations, the withdrawal of vision has no measurable effect of any kind on the outcome of conversation. (p. 411).

Fowler and Wackerbarth (1980) studied the comparison of audio conferencing with face-to-face meetings. They found both laboratory and field research support for the comparability of the two methods for information exchange, discussion of ideas, problem solving, some negotiations, and interviewing. However, they did identify an additional body of research indicating some weaknesses in audio conferencing for certain tasks. Tasks which are of a complex nature, or which involve interpersonal factors may not be suitable for audio conferencing. Thus, it appears that the telephone is an effective substitute for face to face communication in acquiring health information.

The most common use of the telephone for health information is to call the doctor to discuss symptoms. This traditional use of the telephone has been expanded to include hotlines that offer counseling, such as suicide prevention services; dial access services, such as Tel-Med; and information/referral services, such as the Cancer Information Service and related regional services such as the Cancer Lifeline in Seattle.

A small number of the studies which examine the telephone as a medium of health communication focus on the use of the telephone in a physician's practice (Weingarten, 1982; Brown, Helling, Burns, Burmeister, and Rakel, 1982). Five to twenty percent of all patient care contacts are made by telephone (Brown, et al., 1982) and in a pediatric practice, approximately one eighth of the doctors' time is spent in consultation by telephone (Weingarten, 1982). Most of this research seeks to identify the characteristics of the callers, the subjects they call about, and the timing of the calls, with the purpose of better management of a physician's practice. Singer (1981) did examine patients' satisfaction with these telephone contacts and generally found high satisfaction, although a minority of patients complained of being required to speak with a surrogate for their physician such as a secretary or nurse. Pope, Yoshioka, and Greenlick (1971) discovered a greater tendency for more sophisticated individuals to be willing to use the telephone for reporting symptoms to doctors than less sophisticated individuals.

A larger number of studies looked at crisis counseling on the telephone. (e.g., Carothers and Inslee, 1974; Wark, 1982). It has been estimated that the number of emergency hot lines independent of other health and product information services is between 600 and 1000 (Carothers and Inslee, 1974; Rosenbaum and Calhoun, 1977). It is not surprising that so little research has been done on these services. The confidential nature of the calls has forced investigators to explore alternative research strategies, such as analysis of volunteer logbooks and role-playing calls. Most of these alternative research strategies have not been very successful.

Telephone Health Information and Referral Services

Telephone health information and referral services consist of two types: dial-access services such as Tel-Med, which allow callers to request the playing of any of 250 pre-recorded messages on such health subjects as smoking cessation, venereal disease, and arthritis; and interactive services such as the CIS, where trained staff answer questions and refer callers to local resources. Many of the dial-access services are locally developed, often in hospitals. Bartlett, Johnston, and Meyer (1973) report on such a service available at four Madison, Wisconsin hospitals which enables patients to receive audio recordings of four to five minute messages related to the hospital and its personnel, diagnostic procedures, general medical subjects, x-ray studies, and financial matters.

One dial-access service specifically related to cancer is Can-Dial, (Wilkinson, Mirand and Graham, 1985) developed by the Roswell Park Memorial Institute in Buffalo, New York. An individual wanting to use the system dials the advertised number and tells the operator which of the 51 taped messages he/she wishes to hear. The operator loads and plays the selected tape,and an electronic signal at the end of each message shuts off the tape player and breaks the telephone connection.

An interactive information/referral service such as the Cancer Information Service is considerably different from these dial-access services. In fact, we argue that it is a communications system rather than an information system. Dervin (1976) distinguishes between the two in the following way:

> The former (information system) collects, stores, retrieves, and delivers information. The latter (communication system) . . . would help people inform themselves, create their own order, establish their own understandings, and cope with their own accidents. (p. 333).

When using the CIS, the callers define their individual information needs and a knowledgeable staff member gives a personalized response or does research and calls back with the answers. Written material is often sent to the caller as supplementary information. More details about the operation of the CIS are presented in the next chapter.

Data from the CIS have been analyzed in a few previous studies (e.g., Mettlin, et al., 1980; Kramer, et al., 1981; Eckert, 1983), but none of this research used as extensive a data set as the one reported in this book.

New Media

Another way of allowing people to meet their own cancer information needs has been to vary delivery means as well as content. The new interactive format, where the computer acts as a message control device, has been offerred as one solution (Evans and Clarke, 1983). A variety of media for informational display, such as audio tape, frames on conventional television monitors, and segments stored on videodiscs can be used on this type of system.

Another innovative use of these new interactive media is the proposal for a Personal Health Information System (PHIS) (McDonald, 1986). The PHIS would use many media such as printed material, audiotex, video, videotex, microcomputer-based software, and interactive video to deliver quality health information and tools for decision-making. The comprehensive PHIS would have eight major functions:

1. self screening;
2. self assessment;
3. triage;
4. self management;
5. referrals;
6. self exploration;
7. education;
8. personal health planning. (McDonald, 1986, p.4).

It is anticipated that the process of using interactive media may begin to confer self-confidence and a sense of control. Patients can choose a segment, pause when necessary, replay a segment, and take self-administered tests. Unfortunately these innovative health information systems are currently untested and unavailable to most patients.

Summary

This chapter focused on the process used by the public as it seeks health information. Information is defined as some unknown combination of information about reality and information that is the creative product of people. Information has value only in so far as it helps the individual to make sense out of reality.

The health information acquisition process described in our model consists of the following six steps: (1) stimulus; (2) information goal setting; (3) cost/benefit analysis of searching; (4) search behavior; (5) information evaluation; and (6) decision point on adequacy of information.

Sources of health information were categorized using the communication typology of intrapersonal, interpersonal, and mass mediated. Intrapersonal sources include the set of internal knowledge, beliefs, and attitudes about health as well as concrete body sensations. Interpersonal sources include people from whom advice or support is solicited, such as health professionals, family, friends, neighbors, co-workers, acquaintances, and fellow patients. Mass mediated sources include print sources such as newspapers, magazines, and patient education materials, and broadcast sources such as radio, television, telephones, and new communication media. Each of these sources has its own strengths and limitations. Intrapersonal communication is a culmination of all the previous health information seeking experiences and strongly influences what further information is needed or will be accepted. If these intrapersonal sources are inaccurate, they can seriously interfere with subsequent information searches. Ironically, the most reliable and potentially influential interpersonal sources are also the least accessible. The most accessible interpersonal sources, family and friends, are heavily used and quite influential. Mass media sources are pervasive and probably communicate most of their health information indirectly through entertainment programs. Mass media are constrained by space and time pressures which can distort the nature of the health information communicated.

2

Comprehensive Health Communication Systems: A Cancer Example

The previous chapter described the general process of health information seeking, including the variety of sources the seeker might use. This chapter singles out one source of health information, a telephone information/referral program, and describes the challenges information disseminators face when developing and operating such a program. In addition to identifying these challenges, we describe the ways the Cancer Information Service has responded to these challenges through its thirteen year evolution.

The first challenge concerns the nature of the health problem itself. For the CIS, this challenge is a difficult one because cancer is a complex set of diseases which are greatly feared by the public.

The Complexity of Communication About Cancer

We hear a lot about cancer. The news media bombard us with headlines such as "No Way to Avoid Cancer-Causing Agents" and "Tap Water Linked to Cancer." Public service announcements on television educate us about the seven warning signs of cancer and urge us to examine our breasts, stop smoking, eat less fat and more fiber. Recently even commercial sponsors such as Kellogg's cereal company promote their products based on cancer prevention claims. All this information does not necessarily produce educated consumers. Instead, consumers are frequently confused and frustrated. For example, the public may feel more hopeful about having some control over cancer risk when they hear the National Cancer Institute's "Good News" Cancer Prevention Awareness

Campaign. These hopes may be dashed quickly when the same media turn around and report studies claiming we are losing the war on cancer.

Unfortunately, for most of us cancer will not remain a distant threat. Three of every four families will experience cancer first hand. A person who discovers a cancer symptom or is a newly diagnosed cancer patient encounters an even more confusing world full of terms like metastasis, radiation therapy, chemotherapy, and clinical trials. Faced with a myriad of choices, the result may be no action taken or action taken too late to maximize chances for survival and cure. We know, for example, that many people with symptoms wait from three months to a year before they see a physician. Even many of those who begin cancer treatment drop out before completing it.

Few discussions of cancer begin without a litany of the magnitude of its effect on the United States population:

1. About 30 percent of the people living today, or some 74 million people, will eventually have cancer.
2. It is the leading cause of death from disease in children ages 3–14.
3. In 1987 an estimated 965,000 new cases of cancer were diagnosed, *not including* non-melanoma skin cancers (estimated 500,000 cases) and carcinoma in-situ of the cervix.
4. An estimated 483,000 people died of cancer in 1987.
5. One out of every five deaths from *all* causes is from cancer.
6. The age-adjusted mortality rates for cancer have steadily risen from 143 deaths per 100,000 population in 1930 to 170 deaths per 100,000 population in 1984. (American Cancer Society, 1987).

The sheer numbers alone indicate an enormous problem. However, the statistics do not begin to reflect the true impact of cancer in human terms. Cancer is often a fatal disease or accompanied by pain and disfigurement. Cancer patients and their loved ones almost always experience major disruption in their economic, social, and personal lives. Some of the effects of the disease are quite direct, such as the economic cost of treatment, loss of life or limb, pain associated with the disease, and side-effects often associated with its treatment. Other effects are far more subtle, yet no less devastating in their impact: the interruption of a "normal" social life and personal relationships, the loss of sexual identity and "attractiveness" associated with the treatment of certain cancers, the psychological effects of coping with a potentially life threatening situation, and the sense of helplessness and anguish of watching a loved one cope with cancer. The list of ways in which cancer might affect patients and their loved ones is endless. The point, however, is that cancer affects large numbers of the population with devastating, multiple, and varied outcomes that extend beyond the patient to include the individuals and groups who make up the social environment in which he/she participates.

The information presented in the previous paragraphs paints a dismal picture of the extent to which this disease disrupts the lives of those who have it and those who love and care for them. It would not be correct, however, to imply that all the news about cancer is bad. With the allocation of significant funds for research under the National Cancer Act of 1971 and the generous support of organizations such as the American Cancer Society, the Leukemia Society of America, and many others, major strides in cancer prevention, control, and treatment have been made.

Today there are more than 5 million Americans alive who have been cancer patients. In the 1930s, less than 20 percent of cancer patients had any likelihood of surviving for more than 5 years (American Cancer Society, 1987). Data available from the National Cancer Institute indicates that today's 5-year relative survival rate has risen to 49 percent for all sites, sexes and races combined. For the U.S. white population the survival rate is now 50 percent and for children ages 0–14, the rate is 61 percent (NCI, 1987).

In addition to these positive trends, both the National Cancer Institute and the American Cancer Society believe that many more lives could be saved, even without additional research advances. That is, people are dying or suffering today who should not be, given our current knowledge of cancer prevention and control opportunities. The Federal Government's General Accounting Office concluded that a large percentage of cancer patients have not received state-of-the-art cancer treatments for which they were eligible.

> As of 1985, state-of-the-art cancer treatments were not being used in 36.9% of eligible breast cancer patients, 94% of colon cancer patients, 25% of small-cell lung cancer patients, 60% of rectum cancer patients, 50% of nonseminoma testis cancer patients, 18% of patients with Hodgkin's disease, and 20.2% of patients with non-Hodgkin's lymphoma. (Breakthrough Cancer Treatments . . . , 1988, p. 2).

Unique Problems of Communicating About Cancer

Cancer is Highly Feared

Cancer is a fear arousing subject that carries a major connotation of death. The word itself has been used as a metaphor for an evil, invincible predator (Sontag, 1977). One still encounters situations in which people would just as soon not know anything about the subject, particularly if the focus of the discussion is their own risk of the disease.

Messages Vary According to Type of Cancer

The word "cancer" is a term used to describe more than 100 different diseases all characterized by the uncontrolled growth of abnormal cells. Symptoms, methods of detection, treatment, survival rates, and many other aspects of these diseases vary widely among cancer types. Even within a particular type of cancer and often within its clinical stages or progressions, there is professional disagreement on the treatment of choice. Finally, progress in treating cancer varies from type to type. For example, remarkable improvements in survival rates for breast cancer, Hodgkin's disease, and many of the childhood cancers have occurred in the last ten years. On the other hand, the outlook for lung, pancreatic, and liver cancers is still very poor. All of this serves to identify a key problem facing the health communicator: there is no one message to be conveyed when discussing cancer. In fact, there are literally hundreds of different messages which might be desirable to convey.

Messages Encourage Behaviors That are Not Rewarding

The two major message themes for a behavior-oriented communications effort—prevention and early detection—are not very palatable for intended audiences. Obviously, if the problem is one as devastating as cancer, primary prevention would be the ideal theme for a communications effort. Unfortunately, outside of smoking prevention and cessation, some emerging dietary guidelines, and certain techniques for reducing occupational exposure to carcinogens, little practical guidance for the public in terms of the primary prevention of cancer is available. Therefore, the main message in cancer communications is often early detection. This message is based on the improved survival rates and less radical treatment regimens usually associated with the detection of a cancer in its early stages of growth.

The communicator is faced with a dilemma: the message to be conveyed is to adopt behaviors that lead to the early detection of cancer. From the public's perspective, however, the immediate reward for such behavior is negative. That is, to succeed one must find a cancer, submit to a therapy which may be unpleasant, and undergo the associated personal and social trauma of having the disease. Many theories of behavior change recognize that an individual needs to perceive some benefit before adopting a new behavior. With cancer, the immediate, but negative reward, may offset any potential long term benefits.

Messages Face Competition

Cancer communicators also must face competing influences for the public's attention, because cancer is only one of many special health interests. It must compete with multiple other attention-getters, many of which are more attractive and appealing subjects to the public. Also, within the cancer field itself, there are competing messages. Several years ago when interferon was introduced in human clinical trials the media devoted widespread attention to this potential "magic bullet" to cure cancer. At the same time, cautious clinicians and scientists were trying to convey to the public that these were only "trials" and as yet no evidence existed on the efficacy of interferon in treating human cancer. Nevertheless, public desire for a cancer cure, coupled with the media attention devoted to interferon, resulted in raised hopes and appeals for participation in the trials by many more patients than could be admitted or were appropriate candidates.

Finally, cancer communicators face competition in the form of direct opposition to their messages. Despite a ban on cigarette advertising on radio and television, the tobacco industry in this country spends millions of dollars each year in effective advertising for its products. The messages are in direct competition with the cancer communicator's messages based on the premise that 30 percent of all cancer mortality is attributable to smoking. On a similar level, those who wish to prey on the misfortunes of cancer patients spend much time countering conventional cancer therapy messages with those offering easy and painless "cures" for cancer, at a price.

Content of Messages is Constantly Changing

The body of knowledge related to cancer is dynamic and constantly changing. With the tremendous increase in Federal support for cancer research over the last two decades, there has been a corresponding increase in new information available on many aspects of the disease. For the communicator, this expanding body of information creates a continuing need to provide new information as it becomes available. Thus, while there are some standard messages related to cancer (e.g., the importance of early detection), the wide range of new information available presents a challenge to communicators to keep the public updated, without creating a sense of confusion and chaos in their mind.

Messages Vary Across Different Audiences

The important messages to be conveyed about cancer are not the same for all population subgroups. For example, cancer incidence rates over the last several decades show that blacks have higher rates than whites for certain types of cancer, and that the mortality rates may be higher even in those cases where incidence rates are similar. Similarly, rates of skin cancer due to sun exposure are higher for fair-skinned people than for those with darker skins, and higher in people in occupations such as farming, where exposure to sunlight is high, than in those whose occupations do not expose them to sunlight for extended periods.

Cancer is generally a disease of older people and is often assumed to have a long latency period before clinical evidence of disease appears. Thus, it is hard to discuss the subject with younger people who are in the best position to develop sound preventive or early detection habits. In other words, the subject has little relevance to that segment of the population one might most wish to affect.

Relative Risk is Difficult to Convey

The concept of relative risk, a difficult concept to convey in simple terms, is not well understood by the general public interested in decreasing their cancer risks. The problem the communicator faces is that it is virtually impossible to define any specific individual's risk of cancer. Instead, risk is defined in comparative terms derived from group data (e.g., women whose mothers had breast cancer are more likely to get breast cancer than women whose mothers did not). However, everyone seems to know someone who is an exception to any of these general guidelines. The classic example is the person who has smoked heavily for many years and has never developed lung cancer. Thus, cancer risk is difficult to personalize, making it harder to convey a sense of personal relevance to the individual members of the public.

Related to the concept of relative risk is the issue of dose-response relationships in exposure to carcinogens. For example, cigarette smoking is definitely bad for you, but how much worse are four packs a day than two? Very little hard data exist on whether "more is worse" in exposure to carcinogens. Thus, the communicator faces the challenge of dealing with issues of exposure while the determination of whether there is a "safe threshhold" has not yet been made.

Sometimes No Positive Messages Exist

For some cancers there are no positive messages to convey. As noted earlier, for liver and pancreatic cancers there is virtually nothing known about prevention, and while much data are available on treatment, these cancers are rarely detected at a stage when anything can be done for them. That these tumors are in the minority in terms of their relative incidence does not offset the general impression that their high mortality rates convey to the public. Their dismal prognosis contributes to the myth that cancer is a hopeless disease and a sure death sentence.

The Cancer Information Service

Recognizing the enormous information needs that a complex disease such as cancer stimulates, the National Cancer Institute (NCI) in 1975 established a comprehensive communication system, called the Cancer Information Service (CIS). See Appendix A for detailed information on the history and development of the CIS program. The CIS relies on multiple communication media to stimulate and subsequently satisfy cancer information needs. Information on cancer prevention, risk factors, symptoms, detection, treatment, and rehabilitation is provided on a person-to-person basis over the telephone by trained staff members. The CIS handles over 400,000 calls each year from the public through a national telephone number, 1-800-4-CANCER.

The CIS network consisted of 25 regional offices in 1988, serving over 85 percent of the U.S. population. (See Figure 2.1 for those states covered by a regional CIS office.) Appendix B lists all CIS offices. Most offices cover a single state or large population area (e.g., Colorado, New York City). Some offices cover several states (e.g., Florida and Georgia). A national office handles inquiries from remaining areas and provides nationwide coverage after hours and on weekends. Each regional office collects information for and maintains an extensive set of directories on

Cancer Information Service
Regional Offices

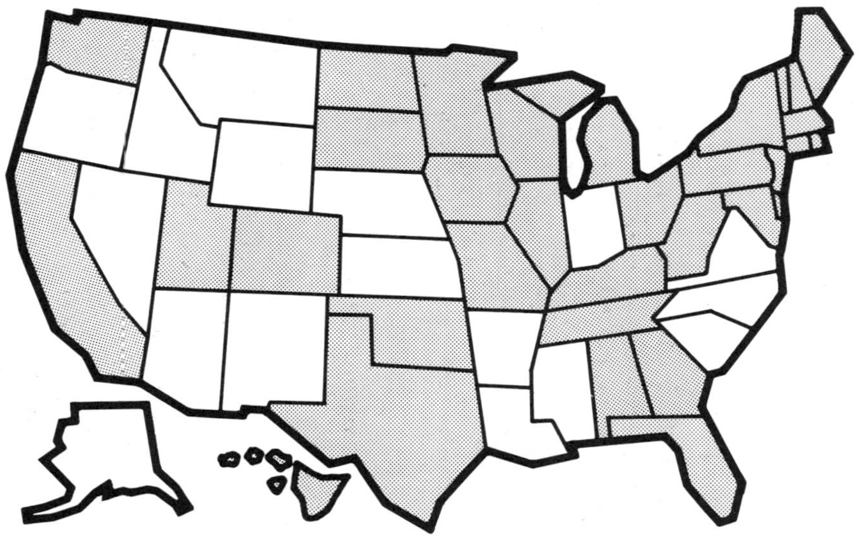

Figure 2.1

cancer-related resources in their service area. Physicians and other health professionals located at regional cancer centers serve as consultants to provide the offices with advice as needed. In addition, each CIS office is routinely provided with information by the NCI reflecting new research and program developments. This information is provided through weekly mailings, daily interaction via an electronic mail system and access to a computerized database developed by NCI. The offices are administered by health communications specialists with an advisory committee providing recommendations on program activities and plans.

The CIS is unique as a resource for health information. It serves the gatekeeping function of gathering, evaluating, selecting, and translating information into a form consumers can comprehend. It provides an immediate, no cost interpersonal source where knowledgeable staff can give personalized responses to questions that anonymous consumers have framed themselves. Most of the health information dissemination efforts studied in the past are campaigns originating from a centralized source and advocating a specific health behavior change. Because the information being disseminated through the CIS is defined by the consumer rather than by a change agent, the CIS is more capable of meeting individual information needs as these needs change over time. Information alone does not necessarily result in improved health practices, but it is an important initial step in health behavior change.

The CIS has become a model program, now being emulated by others in this country and abroad. In the sections that follow we examine the operation of the CIS to identify issues which must be addressed by any comprehensive communications system and to describe the way the CIS has responded to these issues.

The Gatekeeping Role of a Communication System

Questions on a topic as broad as cancer can range from very basic to highly technical, and sources can range from as credible as the *New England Journal of Medicine* to as sensational as checkout line tabloids. Moreover, much of the available literature is too technical and full of medical jargon to be understood by the average person. The challenge in this situation is how to provide comprehensible, accurate, and up-to-date, information on such a broad topic as cancer.

The CIS has responded to this challenge by combining a national and regional set of information resources. Even though the NCI does provide standardized responses to common questions and a variety of consumer materials, it does not limit CIS resources to these institutionally sanctioned publications. The regional offices are encouraged to supplement these national resources with any local information available. The following descriptions of information resources used by the CIS demonstrate how the gatekeeping function can be performed at both centralized and decentralized levels of the system.

National Information Resources

The NCI prepares fact sheets, research reports, pamphlets, and other literature on a wide variety of topics related to cancer. In many cases, answers to callers' questions may be found in these materials, all of which undergo a rigorous review process before publication. Quantities of these materials are on hand in each regional office to use as reference and to mail to callers. NCI also provides CIS offices with access to Physician Data Query (PDQ), a computerized information database described later in this chapter.

In addition, NCI provides each office with a *Standard Response Book* which contains prepared responses to general questions on a variety of cancer topics. CIS staff may quote directly from this book or use the information contained in it to formulate responses if necessary.

A weekly mailing, called the "Weekly Package," is provided to each CIS office by NCI. This package contains newly-developed NCI printed materials, articles from the popular press from the preceding week, relevant scientific articles, and a variety of other items. If one regional office wishes to send printed information to all other offices, it may submit multiple copies for inclusion in this weekly package. The materials distributed may even include information on a new product or service offered by a commercial vendor. All offices understand that inclusion of material in the weekly package does not imply NCI endorsement of a particular product or service, but information of this nature is often useful in responding to the callers' needs.

Regional Information Resources

Since the regionalization of the CIS is a key feature of the program, each field office is responsible for compiling and continuously updating a resource directory for its service area. This directory normally covers resources in at least one state. The questions from callers cover the continuum of cancer, ranging from the general public's concern about screening or prevention through the needs of people with symptoms for diagnostic testing and the needs of patients for support groups, medical equipment, or rehabilitation services. Therefore, the CIS resource directories contain listings of the following types of resources in order to be responsive to all callers' needs. Information collected on each of the community resources generally includes cost, referral information (e.g., eligibility requirements), hours of operation, and a description of the services provided.

- Hospitals and clinics treating cancer, with notation of their special capabilities, interests, equipment, etc.
- Cancer screening programs by cancer site including breast and cervical screening as well as general cancer screening programs.
- Self-help programs for cancer patients (e.g., ostomy or laryngectomy groups).
- Regional office listings for voluntary agencies concerned with cancer, such as the American Cancer Society, and the services provided by each.
- Materials, services and educational programs available from cancer-concerned organizations.
- Non-cancer-oriented organizations providing services useful to cancer patients and/or their families (e.g. transportation, blood banks).
- Sources of financial and legal assistance.
- Employment and training opportunities.
- Professional organizations related to cancer.
- Medical supply agencies.
- Nursing services.
- Prevention oriented activities, e.g., worksite health promotion programs and risk reduction programs.
- Counseling sources, including smoking cessation programs.

It is important to note that although the offices keep track of the types of organizations and services noted above, they do not hold themselves responsible for the services actually provided. A disclaimer is offered to callers indicating that while the CIS has compiled this information, it has been provided by the organizations themselves. Although attempts are made to verify the existence and quality of services, the CIS has never assumed the role of endorsing services or comparing the value of one program or service to another.

Each office maintains a library of appropriate medical and other textbooks for reference purposes, as well as popular press books on cancer.

In many cases, callers need clarification of medical terminology, descriptions of diagnostic or surgical procedures, or other basic scientific and medical information contained in these texts.

Information materials of a changing nature are generally kept in vertical files which undergo regular updating. These files might include newspaper clippings on specific topics, pamphlets produced by various non-NCI or CIS organizations, and scientific articles. Each office establishes a system to determine which material in these files is to be used for internal purposes only (usually a newspaper clipping will fall into this category) and which materials may be used to directly respond to callers' questions. This information is usually stamped according to whether or not it may be quoted from or mailed to callers.

Access to needed resources is of critical importance in the operation of information dissemination systems such as the CIS. Without the continuous gathering, sorting, and updating necessary to maintain these resources, the ability to respond to the ever-changing nature of the public's information needs is diminished.

Staffing a Comprehensive Communication System

The key to the success of any large-scale communication system is the quality of the staff who interact directly with its users. Some of the challenges surrounding staffing a system are: determining the functions which staff must perform, deciding whether to use volunteer or paid staff, training the staff, and maintaining quality control of responses given by the staff. The key staff in each regional CIS office include those described below.

Necessary Staff Functions

Program advisor/advocate

This person is usually a high-ranking professional in the parent institution who serves 5–10 percent time on the CIS program (in the CIS program, the parent institution is generally a cancer center which is part of a large medical institution or university-based medical school). He/she usually serves the function of program advisor and advocate, representing the CIS to higher-ups in the organizational structure.

Program manager

This person usually holds a full-time position, providing overall program management and coordination, and fulfills reporting requirements both to the parent institution and to NCI. The program manager is usually responsible for staff recruitment and hiring, publicity and promotion, quality control and evaluation, and representation of the CIS program to its many constituents. People serving as CIS managers come from a wide variety of backgrounds with degrees, often advanced, in such fields as public health, communications, allied medical specialties (e.g., nursing, social work), and the social sciences. Management skills are essential for this position, as well as excellent oral and written communication skills.

Telephone supervisor

This full-time position has overall responsibility for operation of the CIS telephone service, including staff training, day to day supervision, and maintenance of information resources. A medical or social service background is helpful for effective communication about the complex topic of cancer to other staff as well as to callers. These positions are often held by people with training in allied medical fields as well as supervisory skills.

Information specialists

These staff respond directly to public inquiries. The staffing needs for these positions are dependent upon the size of the population served by the office. On the average, an office serving a population area from 1–5 million will require 2.5 full-time information specialists. Three or more information specialists are required if the population served is larger than this. Responding to telephone inquiries can be a very demanding and stressful job, and many offices have hired multiple part-time information specialists to supplement or in lieu of full-time individuals. If full-time staff are utilized, it is helpful to intersperse telephone duties with other assignments, such as resource updating and maintenance. These positions are well suited to individuals with health and/or counseling backgrounds.

Evaluation specialist

Since CIS data must be tabulated regularly, it must be entered into machine-readable format. This position is usually 30–40 percent time, depending upon the number of inquiries handled. Some offices choose to sub-contract this function to a data-processing firm.

Secretary

One full-time secretary is needed to handle the clerical responsibilities of each office.

Paid Staff Versus Volunteers

Volunteers are attractive sources of inexpensive labor for many low-budget communication systems. Although several CIS offices are still utilizing volunteers successfully, others that previously used volunteers to help staff the office are now relying totally on paid staff. Among the reasons cited for this decision are the following:

- The caliber of volunteer needed to respond to complex inquiries is quite high. Many individuals with the background and skills necessary to perform the job of CIS information specialist are usually in the workforce themselves and not seeking volunteer positions.
- Many volunteers are only interested in serving for a limited number of hours each week. Because of the need to keep current with rapidly changing information, minimum weekly time commitments are required (e.g., eight hours/week), which often cannot be met by volunteers.
- Some volunteers are only able to serve for a limited length of time, e.g., students during a one-semester placement. The amount of time needed to train and orient these individuals almost can equal their total time commitment in the office.
- The amount of paid staff time required for volunteer recruitment, training, scheduling, and day to day supervision may be equal to or greater than the time the volunteers actually provide to the office. Thus, it may be more efficient to replace these volunteer "maintenance" functions and utilize paid staff to respond to the inquiries themselves.

A careful assessment of staffing needs and access to qualified volunteers will help determine if their use is appropriate for other comprehensive communications systems.

Staff Training

In order for the staff of a comprehensive health communications program to disseminate accurate, timely, and appropriate information to callers, they must have extensive, systematic, and continuous training. Initially, staff training for the CIS was the responsibility of each regional office. By 1980, the need was recognized for a comprehensive, standardized training program that could be used by all offices. A task force working with NCI staff developed a standardized training curriculum for use throughout the CIS network of regional offices. It recommends a 36-hour didactic program for each staff member, followed by experience in listening to inquiries handled by trained staff members, role-playing typical call scenarios, oral examinations, practice calls, and calls taken with the supervisor listening to the conversation. It should be pointed out that ALL staff in each office regardless of their positions are required to complete the initial staff training program, and are required to serve a minimum of two hours per week responding to CIS inquiries. This requirement assures that CIS staff at all levels can handle inquiries if needed (e.g., when a news story generates a large number of calls during a short period of time). In addition, it is felt that routinely staffing the telephone lines aids the CIS management staff in staying "in touch" with the public's information needs.

In addition to using the standard training program for new staff members, each office is required to develop a program of ongoing staff training and professional development. This program includes an annual refresher training course to review operating procedures and basic cancer concepts and information; a continuing education program of at least four hours each three months on cancer-related topics of current public, media or research interest; and other training as needed. Staff are also encouraged to attend and participate in seminars and other educational opportunities offered through their parent institution or other organizations.

On occasion, NCI develops additional training curricula in response to particular needs. Several years ago, it became apparent that CIS offices were not well equipped to provide counseling to callers who wished to quit smoking. An extensive training program was developed and one staff member from each regional office came to NCI for a "train-the-trainers" session. In turn, they trained the remainder of the staff on smoking cessation counseling.

Promotion

Promotion of a health communications system is critically important. If the public do not know of the program's existence, they cannot use it. Moreover, promotion must be continuous since people's information needs will change if they move along the disease continuum from general public to symptomatic to patient. When national and regional offices are involved, responsibility for promotion must be determined.

The CIS experienced difficulty promoting the service in the first few years because of the need to include different telephone numbers for each office. With the availability of a single "800" number, NCI staff working with a CIS task force developed a promotion plan based on social marketing techniques (Sciandra and Stein, 1983). More detailed promotion information will be presented in Chapter Eight.

In recent years, program promotion has been steady, with planned campaigns developed to reach specific target audiences. The press routinely places the CIS telephone number in cancer-related articles. News events that temporarily flood telephone lines still occasionally occur, such as President Reagan's colon cancer, diagnosed in 1985 (discussed further in Chapter Eight). In these cases the CIS telephone number is offered to all callers from the media so that the public will know how to find additional information. Promotion of the CIS has been so effective that it may be said the CIS has become a "victim of its success," as seen by the increasing number of inquiries each year. (See Figure 2.2) A limited number of incoming telephone lines and staff enable a finite number of callers to reach the CIS at any one time, leading to caller frustration. Although innovations in communication technology (described later in this chapter) have aided in making the CIS more efficient, those directing any comprehensive communications system must be cognizant of the results that may be generated from successful promotion campaigns and plan accordingly.

Number of Inquiries by Year
Cancer Information Service

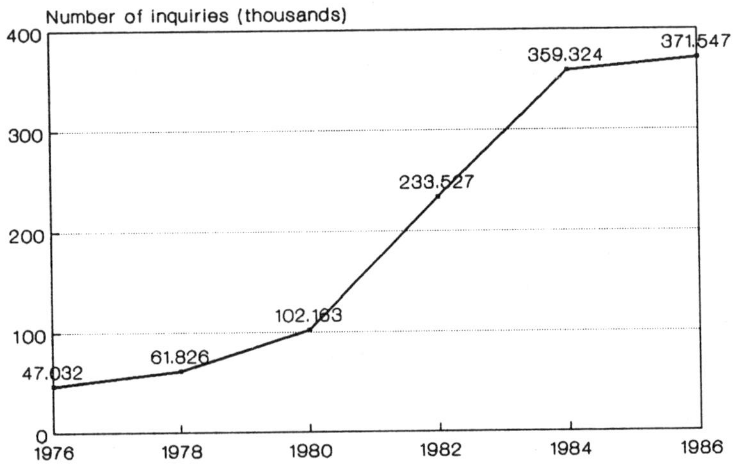

Figure 2.2

Evaluation

The importance of evaluation for any health communications program cannot be overstated. Evaluation can and should be used as a means of determining whether program goals and objectives are being accomplished, and as a management tool to continually assess and improve service delivery. The CIS struggled for several years before formulating a national evaluation plan. A three-part evaluation has been used for the past five years: a standardized call record form which documents several characteristics of each call; a user survey which assesses satisfaction with the service; and the quality control program designed to monitor the performance of the information specialists. The first two are sources of the data presented in this book and will be described in more detail in the next chapter. The quality control program will be described in a following section.

The longevity of the CIS has depended to a large extent on the results of this national evaluation. In the late 1970s and the early 1980s, the CIS was heavily criticized as too expensive with too little data to demonstrate its accomplishments. When approval was reluctantly given by NCI's scientific advisors in 1982 to extend the program an additional three years until 1985, it was clear that solid measures of its accomplishments would be a prerequisite for any further extensions of the funding. When the initial evaluation data were presented in 1984, the same group of scientific advisors gave the program their enthusiastic support.

In addition to its accountability function, evaluation has been invaluable for program management. Evaluation data enable offices to track call volume in ways that allow for more rational staffing patterns to evolve; to track public response to specific promotion or media events; to monitor the effects of new technology; and to compare data among offices that provide a basis for technical advice and consultation.

Quality Control

Quality control is a critical aspect of any information program. If the response given to an inquiry is not reliable or useful, the program cannot possibly accomplish its desired objectives. For the CIS the issue of quality control is a particularly difficult one to deal with. First of all, as noted elsewhere in this chapter, cancer is a highly complex set of diseases and the potential range of questions that might be asked about them is enormous. Furthermore, the knowledge base used to answer questions is constantly changing and expanding due to new research findings. Finally, because the CIS is a network of multiple regional offices consisting of hundreds of employees and volunteers who respond to inquiries, the problem of quality control is compounded by having so many "points-of-contact." For the most part, CIS has been gifted with dedicated and capable staff for whom quality control has been perceived as a natural and necessary part of their jobs. Nevertheless, to manage effectively a large and complicated program such as this requires a formal plan and procedures for quality assurance.

The first step in designing a quality control plan was to define a set of "quality control dimensions" that could be applied to any telephone inquiry.

CIS dimensions of quality

A. Accuracy

- **1.** Correct—Information is contained within NCI-produced materials or, depending upon the question, a recognized and appropriate non-NCI reference may be used (for example, American Cancer Society publications).
- **2.** Timely—Information given is from the most recently produced sources.
- **3.** Complete—Not missing any standard information given by recognized sources.
- **4.** Precise—Not encumbered by extra or irrelevant information.

B. Convenience

- **1.** Accessible—A CIS staff member is readily available. If not readily available, an explanation is offered.
- **2.** Prompt—In most cases, the information needed to answer the question is readily at hand. In cases where further research is necessary, an explanation will be offered and the CIS staff member will ask the caller to phone again or offer to return the call when the information is obtained.

C. Appropriateness

- **1.** Responsive—Information offered is that which will respond to all questions asked.
- **2.** Referrals—Referrals (if indicated) are responsive to the questions asked by the caller.
- **3.** Language—Language appropriate to the situation is used, including explanations of medical terminology and acronyms or other jargon.

D. Staff Sensitivity

- **1.** Empathetic—Perceived ability of CIS staff to take the perspective of the caller.

2. Friendly—CIS staff member is perceived as kind, not hostile towards the caller.
3. Credible—CIS staff member conveys a sense of authority and competence in delivering the response.

E. Effectiveness
Behavior—Information given by the CIS resulted in appropriate behavior (if indicated) on the part of the caller.

F. Standardization
1. Intra-center—Callers asking the same question handled by different staff in the same office are given the same general answer.
2. Inter-center—Callers asking the same question of staff at different offices are given the same general answer.

With the dimensions of quality defined for the CIS network, the next step in developing a quality control plan was to determine the means by which they could be achieved. For the most part, quality control for a program like CIS is dependent on the resources available to respond to inquiries, the type of staff recruited and their maintenance and retention, the training that staff receives at the outset and throughout their period of service, and the quality of the supervision and guidance staff receive from program managers.

The major challenge for NCI staff related to quality control then became monitoring it. Recognizing that the real means of quality control would always be most evident at the "point-of-contact" when a caller asked a question of a CIS staff member, a test call system was developed which attempted to approximate actual operating conditions for a CIS. With this system, periodic test calls are placed from NCI staff located in Bethesda, Maryland to staff in each office. The telephone company has provided numbers through which each local WATS line can be directly accessed, thus making the test calls appear as a regular call to the local office's number. A standardized approach to doing test calls was developed after some trial and error (Stein and Kean, 1982). Test call scenarios with questions and minimum expected responses are developed by NCI staff and approved by appropriate clinical and scientific staff at the NCI. In addition to developing the questions and answers, standardized background information (e.g., age, medical history) is developed for each call, so that the test caller can respond to probing on the part of the CIS information specialists.

In general, one person places the call, while another person listens to the conversation on another telephone and takes extensive notes. Standard rating scales for each of the quality dimensions noted earlier are prepared and filled out immediately after the test call by both the person placing the call and the person listening to the call. Test calls are prepared and delivered periodically in such a way that all regional offices receive the same call before going on to a new round of calls on a different question.

To be effective, a quality assurance program must also be prepared to act on the results it finds. As a matter of routine, each regional office is debriefed in writing by the NCI project officer for each test call received. For the most part, responses to test calls are satisfactory or better. However, even in these cases valuable tips for improving services can be provided to staff.

Before implementing the test call system, a series of graduated procedures for corrective action were outlined in the event a less than satisfactory result was achieved by any regional office. At a minimum, if an unsatisfactory response is received during a test call, repeated test calls on different topics are placed over the next several days. If satisfactory results are achieved on these, the only action taken is to notify the local CIS manager of the unsatisfactory call and to discuss its outcome in detail, leaving any further corrective action to be taken at the local level. If additional testing results in more unsatisfactory responses, immediate action is taken to correct the deficiences noted. It is important to note that it has rarely been necessary to take action beyond debriefing, since the general response to test calls is quite good. On one occasion, however, inadequate responses to test calls prompted NCI to require a regional office to switch its phone lines to the national office for a period of two weeks during which its staff were retrained. In that one extreme case, the office was repeatedly retested with test calls for an extended period even after starting up operations again.

Adoption and Use of Communication Technology

A comprehensive health communication system must utilize some form of communication technology to reach its users. The telephone, the technology used by the CIS, has many advantages. It is almost universally available, low-cost, and simple to use. Perhaps most important, it allows a personalized service to be delivered to the public. Moreover, new telephone technology is constantly being developed without increasing the complexity for the individual user. The CIS has adopted many of these innovations. Each of the major technological innovations adopted for the CIS program will be discussed, with a description of the circumstances leading to their adoption and the resulting program impact.

Toll-Free Telephone Lines (WATS Lines)

Toll-free telephone numbers, introduced in this country in 1969, were first widely used by businesses for convenient customer access. In this system, accessed by "800"-prefix telephone numbers, the costs are absorbed by the sponsoring organization rather than the caller. Non-profit organizations were slower to note that convenient access was important to a program's success. For a public service program such as the CIS, user access should be as convenient as possible. It was also felt that users should not incur any charges for telephone access to the program. Therefore, from the beginning of the program, each regional office established toll-free telephone lines for its service area (usually a state or group of states). The cost of the toll-free service has been borne by the NCI, or in some cases, by the parent institution sponsoring the regional office. The CIS national office, which handles calls from areas where no regional office exists, after hours, and on weekends, established additional toll-free lines, accessible from anywhere in the country.

Single Number Service

Although WATS lines enabled convenient access for the user, the system in its original form was impossible to promote effectively. Until 1983, each regional office had a separate toll-free telephone number. When offices covered more than one state, different numbers were needed for each state covered. The total program at that time included thirty-four different toll-free telephone numbers. Each number was only accessible to people calling from within a particular state. Although regional offices could promote the use of their toll-free number within their own service area, this system made national promotion unwieldy. For example, when television public service announcements were developed, a separate "tag" consisting of a slide of the local telephone number had to be prepared for each office. The slide was included with the film or tape, and had to be inserted by public service directors prior to airing the announcement. The extra effort required to use CIS public service announcements diminished their competitiveness with other organizations for air time.

This problem extended to the print media. For the national press to refer readers to the CIS required printing thirty-four separate telephone numbers. Space constraints usually prohibited their use. In addition, these telephone numbers were difficult to remember. The very public CIS wished to serve was often ignorant of its existence or unable to remember the appropriate CIS telephone number.

The solution to these problems came in the form of a telecommunications innovation known as "Expanded 800" service. Through this new service, a single, toll-free telephone number was adopted for the entire CIS program. With this system, calls made to a single number are automatically routed to the appropriate regional office according to the area code from which the call is placed. For example, if the number is dialed in Pennsylvania, it is automatically routed to the CIS office in Philadelphia, which serves that state. When an office serves more than one state, calls are automatically routed to the appropriate office. Thus, the office located in Boston automatically receives calls from Massachusetts, Maine, Vermont, and New Hampshire, all part of its service area. Calls from areas not covered by a regional office are routed to the national CIS office at NCI.

Now that a single number could be promoted, a series of numbers could be chosen that would be both easily recalled and representative of the service offered. Using the letters on the telehone dial to create a mnemonic term seemed the solution. The number, 1-800-4-CANCER (1-800-422-6237), was chosen. Users remember this number, even some time after exposure to it. Promotion of this single number, both locally and nationally, has dramatically increased the number of calls to the CIS. (See Chapter Eight for description of call rates and usage of the single number in promotion.)

Another benefit derived from adoption of this system is that it serves an important program management function. CIS project staff at NCI have control over distribution of calls to regional offices through the "Expanded 800" system. NCI staff can quickly change the office to which calls are automatically routed by notifying telephone company representatives. Therefore, when new offices join the program, calls from their area are rerouted from the national CIS to the new local office. In addition, if there should be a serious problem in one office, it is possible to have calls rerouted to another office either temporarily or permanently. In information programs where quality control in regional offices is an issue, control over the use of the national telephone number can be a "big stick" to use if quality falters in the field or if national program guidelines are not being followed locally.

Triaging Calls

Implementation of the "Expanded 800" service in 1983 increased call rates beyond all expectations. However, it also led to some problems. Offices began to complain of staff burnout from the pressures of responding to an ever-increasing number of telephone inquiries. In addition, the number of callers with simple publication requests, as opposed to specific questions, rose dramatically due to several national promotion campaigns. Between January and June, 1983, 9.5 percent of callers requested specific publications; the number rose to 43.5 percent of callers between July and December, 1984. In general, callers receiving publications increased from 45 percent to 71 percent during this same period. Obviously, much more professional staff time had to be devoted to preparation and assembling of publications to mail. The offices were literally becoming publications warehouses.

Not only was this an inefficient use of professional staff time, but each publication was costing double to mail, once when the publications were sent to the regional offices from the central NCI warehouse, and again when the publications were mailed from the regional offices to the caller. Postage costs began to escalate dramatically.

To make matters worse, studies of call attempts performed by the telephone company in 1984 revealed that an average of 19 percent of calls to all CIS offices were lost due to busy signals. So, not only were offices handling an inordinate number of simple publication requests, but many callers with serious concerns may not have reached CIS offices. With the call rates continuing to increase, it was assumed that busy signals, and therefore lost calls, would also increase. Lost calls were projected to reach 30 percent by 1985, an unacceptable level.

NCI recommended that offices install telephone sequencers as a partial solution to the problem. These devices intercept calls and deliver a recorded message to the caller, asking them to stay on the line until a staff member is free to take the call. This solution was not completely satisfactory. The sequencers only intercept a call if a telephone line is free. In many offices, the lines were in use most of the time. In that case, callers received a busy signal.

Again, the solution to this series of problems came in the form of a telecommunications innovation, called "Advanced 800" service. Adoption of this system in no way affected callers' use of the single, toll-free number. What it did was add a triaging system, whereby a taped message instructs callers to either order publications or ask cancer-related questions by pushing either "one" or "two" on their telephone pad. If they wish to ask questions, pushing "one" will automatically connect them with the regional office serving their area. If they wish simply to order publications, they reach a central publications office which was established to handle publications orders from all parts of the country.

The "Advanced 800" system was implemented throughout the CIS program in 1985. One immediate benefit of the system was economic.

Because calls in each regional office declined by approximately 25 percent with the new central publications ordering service (the POS), a small reduction in staff time was possible in each office. In addition, postage costs for regional offices decreased substantially.

Surprisingly, even though regional offices reported drops in call rates at an average of 25 percent, busy signal studies revealed that the CIS was still losing approximately 20 percent of calls. This busy signal rate may be explained by the more complicated nature of the calls now handled by the program and the fact that the number of staff and the number of telephone lines has remained constant for some time due to budgetary constraints.

Use of the "Advanced 800" also forced changes in promoting the CIS. Previously, many promotions focused on a specific publication, giving the CIS telephone number to order it. Recent promotions have positioned the CIS as a number to call for answers to specific questions, rather than a place to order publications, which has affected the nature of the inquiries. Where previously 24 percent of calls to regional offices were from cancer patients and their families, now these calls average 43 percent of users. Calls from the general public have declined from 57 percent to 34 percent of users. Inquiries about specific cancer sites have increased 37 percent, and the number of callers who have used the service previously is up 12 percent. As expected, publications are now mailed to fewer callers, down 23 percent from previous figures. Also, the amount of time spent on each call has increased, with calls longer than six minutes in length rising from 23 percent to 44 percent of all inquiries.

By eliminating the majority of calls with simple publication requests from regional offices, the pool of likely CIS users has been systematically narrowed to those whom are felt to be most in need. With limited staff and resources, comprehensive communications systems cannot be "all things to all people." It is important to define priority groups and channel efforts accordingly.

Electronic Mail and Bulletin Board

While there are many advantages to a decentralized system with regional offices, the intra-system communications can be quite difficult and complicated. At least twice each week, simultaneous communication with all offices had been needed, for example, to alert them of some fast-breaking news event that might affect their calls (e.g., the CIS telephone number would appear in a national promotion the next morning) or to gather information for management purposes. Until 1986, these needs were met either by mass mailings or by telephone calls to all offices, both of which could take from one-half to a full day of staff time. These necessary but time-consuming communications taxed the small program management staff at NCI.

An electronic mail system was implemented to alleviate this communications problem. Through the use of computer terminals and telephone modems, a central computer is accessed each day by each office in the system. It is possible to send messages to one office, a group of offices, or all offices at once. The message is entered and each person on the system receives it when they access their electronic "mailbox" daily.

This system also includes an electronic bulletin board which provides daily access to cancer-related stories issued by the major wire services and new information disseminated by NCI to the public and health professionals.

Any comprehensive communications system with regional offices would benefit by implementation of a similar system. It is relatively inexpensive because any computer terminal and modem can be used for electronic mail access.

Computerized Information Retreival

Disseminating accurate and timely information on a health issue as complex as cancer requires an ability to access the most up-to-date information available. Sometimes technology has been developed for other purposes which also can be used an an information resource. For example, Physician Data Query (PDQ), a computerized data base providing the most up-to-date cancer treatment information, was originally developed by NCI to disseminate the latest information to physicians. PDQ has become a first-line resource for each CIS office. The information is updated monthly by NCI, thus making it an extremely valuable and timely resource for responding to cancer treatment inquiries. CIS offices have access to the data base on-line, and each office is provided with a hard copy of the cancer treatment information.

From the problems and solutions noted above, it is evident that communications technology can play a critical role in the evolution of a comprehensive health communication program. As new innovations emerge, the program can adopt them to improve efficiency, cost effectiveness, and quality of service.

Summary

This chapter has presented some of the challenges faced in developing and operating a comprehensive health communication system and described how the CIS responded to those challenges. The first challenge discussed was the nature of the health issue itself. Cancer is a particularly difficult communication problem because it is such a complex set of diseases and so highly feared by the public. The CIS was designed as a comprehensive communication system charged with providing accurate, timely, and comprehensible cancer information to the public. The structure of the CIS consists of a set of regional offices, coordinated by the National Cancer Institute, that uses the telephone to link users to information specialists.

The CIS was used as a model to show how a communications system might address such issues as its gatekeeping role, staffing needs, training program, promotion, evaluation, quality control, and use of evolving communication technology.

3

The Cancer Information Service Evaluation: An Overview of Results

Critical to the success of any large-scale communications system is an understanding of its users: who they are, their information needs, their satisfaction with the information provided, and the system's influence on their behavior. In this chapter, we describe standard collection and reporting procedures used in a four-year analysis (1983–86) of all CIS inquiries and a user survey of a subset of this group. We present an overview of results from these two databases.

Data Set and Collection Methods

Description of the Data Collection Form

A call record form (CRF) is completed for every inquiry to the CIS by the person handling that inquiry. The CRF (see example, Appendix C), consists of an 8 1/2" x 14" two-sided form and an accompanying list of codes. Information is written directly onto each form, including a narrative description of the inquiry and response and a number of precoded items.

The CRF collects three types of information from CIS users: administrative, inquiry/response, and user demographics. The administrative information consists of identification data including date, location of CIS office, staff ID number, case number, time taken to handle the call, and follow-up action (e.g., sending pamphlets to callers). Administrative information is recorded consistently for every call.

Inquiry/response data describe the nature and content of the interaction between the caller and CIS staff. A broad range of information is included. The CRF includes 56 categories for "Subject of Inquiry," and up to five codes may be used for each call. For example, questions are often asked regarding specific types and sites of cancer (e.g., Tell me all you can about breast cancer). Callers also may be seeking information about the CIS or other organizations concerned with cancer such as the American Cancer Society or regional cancer centers. They may request referrals for physicians, medical equipment, home care services, and counseling programs. Risk factors may be of concern to callers (e.g., What are the dangers of second hand smoke if you live with a smoker?). Callers may, additionally, ask about available treatments (e.g., How do I find out what new treatment is available for my type of cancer?). All items with the exception of subject of inquiry are generally coded by the individual handling the call and specifically trained individual(s) in each office are responsible for coding the subject of inquiry section on every call.

When information of a medical nature is discussed that has the potential of being applied to individual cases, CIS information specialists give callers a medical disclaimer. The disclaimer, which is printed on the form, may be read or paraphrased, and is worded as follows:

> I have given you our most accurate and up-to-date information. However, you should keep in mind that I am not a medical doctor. If you have requested this information because of your own medical condition or for someone you know, the information I have given you should be discussed with your physician. Only a physician who has a complete medical history of a person can determine what is advisable in that particular case.

Callers also are coded by type (e.g., diagnosed patient, undiagnosed person with symptoms, relative of patient, health professional, student, general public). There are twenty specific caller types, which helps the CIS staff to determine how and why the information is used. For example, health professionals may call for updated information, students for research purposes, and patients for treatment information or referrals for counseling. As a result of a conversation, a staff member may offer behavioral suggestions to the caller. The twenty coded responses for such suggestions include referrals (e.g., NCI, second opinion, counseling/support group), reading mailed literature, and encouraging the practice of self-detection techniques, improved diet, or smoking cessation.

The third type of information recorded is user demographics. These data include age, sex, education, ethnic background, and state location of the caller. Callers are also asked how they first found out about the CIS (e.g., word of mouth, TV, radio, telephone book), and whether they have used the service before. User demographics are important in determining which "audience" is using the CIS and which media are most effective in reaching those callers.

Data Collection Methods

Following development of the call record form (CRF), a four-week pilot test was conducted at three of the CIS offices. An operations manual for the CRF was created and each office introduced the use of the form and trained its phone staff to fill out the CRF properly. Of the 1,803 CRFs coded during the pilot test, a sample of 100 were sent to six individuals to assess the consistency of the coding. A high degree of concurrence was noted in all coding categories except "subject of inquiry," where there was disagreement on the number of codes used for the more complicated inquiries. In 67 percent of the forms coded, at least four of the six individuals were in agreement on the codes assigned. Considering that any one form may have had as many as five different codes assigned out of a pool of 56 coding categories, this level of concurrence is reasonable. However, it should be noted that concurrence is much higher for the analysis reported in this book for two reasons. First, the coding categories were modified following pilot testing, and second, the 56 coding categories have been collapsed into ten broad categories for this analysis. More specific and detailed information on the pilot test and the other data elements were described in a thesis (Ferguson, 1983).

Standard data collection in all offices began on January 1, 1983 and continued uninterrupted through the four-year period of this study. The procedures for the CRF are simple. A form is filled out for all information requests from the public and health professionals, including telephone calls, mail requests, and walk-ins. As noted, in most offices one individual is responsible for assuring all coding is in accordance with the definitions and procedures contained in the operations manual. Data are entered onto a computer tape in a standard format and submitted to NCI each six months. At NCI the data are processed into a single data set and prepared for analysis.

Overview of CIS Calls

Description of the Callers and Their Questions

The analysis upon which this book is based consists of 1,380,925 CIS inquiries made from January, 1983 through December, 1986. In this section, the complete data set will be described briefly, with more extensive analysis of the data to be found in Chapters Four through Seven for the various users of the CIS. Compared to most evaluations, this study has a very large number of cases. As a result, applying standard statistical tests consistently yields differences that are highly significant, but which may or may not be programmatically meaningful. Therefore, we do not report the results of these tests but rather present those trends and comparative differences which have programmatic significance. It also should be noted that the overall data analysis contained in this chapter masks important differences among specific CIS user groups which are discussed in more detail in the next chapter. Later chapters focus on three specific CIS user groups: the general public, symptomatic individuals and their families/friends, and cancer patients and their families/friends.

Almost all CIS inquiries were telephone calls (98%), with less than one percent of the inquiries consisting of face-to-face contact in the CIS office. Nearly 20 percent of inquiries were from previous users of the system. In order to avoid duplication, demographic data (i.e., sex, age, education, and ethnic background) were not collected on previous users.

Who are the Callers?

Type of callers

Each CIS inquiry is classified according to the type of caller, relative to his/her inquiry. For example, a nurse calling about her husband who had cancer would be classified as a family member rather than as a health professional. Members of the general public were the most frequent users of the CIS, accounting for almost 47 percent of all inquiries. (See Figure 3.1.) This category also includes students seeking cancer information for school-related activities (2.1%). Families and friends of cancer patients comprised 22.4 percent of all users. In many instances it appeared that the patient's family and friends act as "health agents," seeking information on a patient's behalf. Cancer patients themselves call much less frequently, accounting for only 11 percent of all calls. Individuals with symptoms and their families and friends accounted for another 8.2 percent of callers. These were people who were inquiring about symptoms

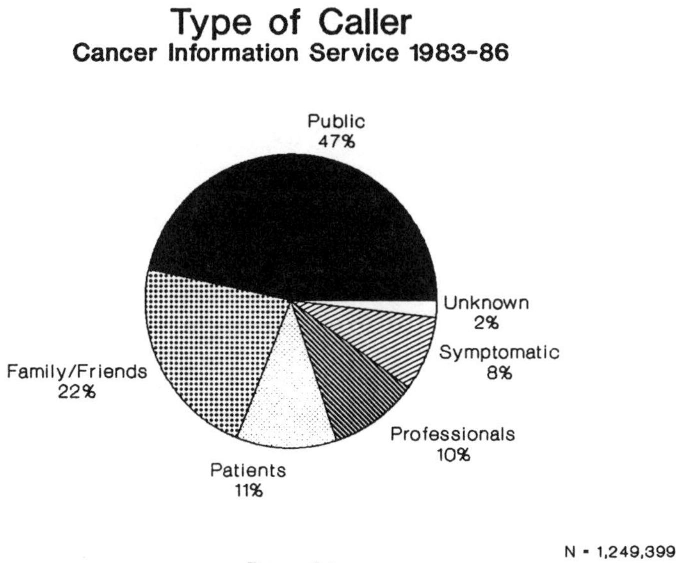

Figure 3.1

that may or may not eventually be diagnosed as cancer, but cause concern to the caller. Health care and other professionals, calling in that capacity, accounted for almost 10 percent of callers. Of those, 2 percent were nurses and 1.4 percent physicians. Other health professionals included social workers, dietitians, pharmacists, educators, the clergy, and representatives of the American Cancer Society (ACS). Others with questions related to their professions included attorneys and insurance agents.

Sex of callers

Females used the CIS much more than males, accounting for 71 percent of all CIS inquiries (Figure 3.2), a much larger proportion than the 51.4 percent of females in the U.S. population. This disproportionate use by females has been consistent over the years, and was a source of some criticism in the program's early years. However, we believe that much of the information gathered by women is passed along to others, including men. Women callers often state that they are asking questions on behalf of their husbands or fathers, and are possibly acting as the "information gatherers" of the family.

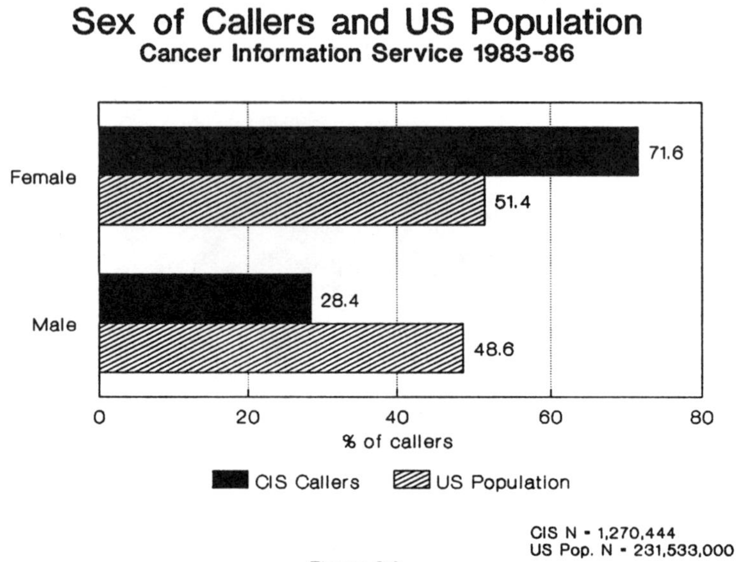

Figure 3.2

Age of callers

Figure 3.3 illustrates the age distribution of CIS callers compared to the 1980 population. In general, CIS callers tend to be older than the overall population; this seems reasonable because cancer incidence increases with age, and interest in the topic may increase as well. The most frequent users of the CIS are in the 30 to 39 age category, followed by users aged 20 to 29. Users in the 40 to 49 and 50 to 59 age groups called more often than their representation in the overall population, and callers aged 60 and over called in the same proportion as their population figures would indicate. Children and teens only account for 8 percent of CIS callers compared to their 30.7 percent share of the U.S. population. These results are expected since they are consistent with the age ranges of people likely to be affected by cancer.

Education level of callers

CIS users also are more educated than the U.S. adult population, as illustrated in Figure 3.4. Over 53 percent of CIS users have at least some college, compared to just over 30 percent of the population. Only 47 percent of CIS users had a high school diploma or less, in contrast with almost 70 percent of the general population. It could be speculated that

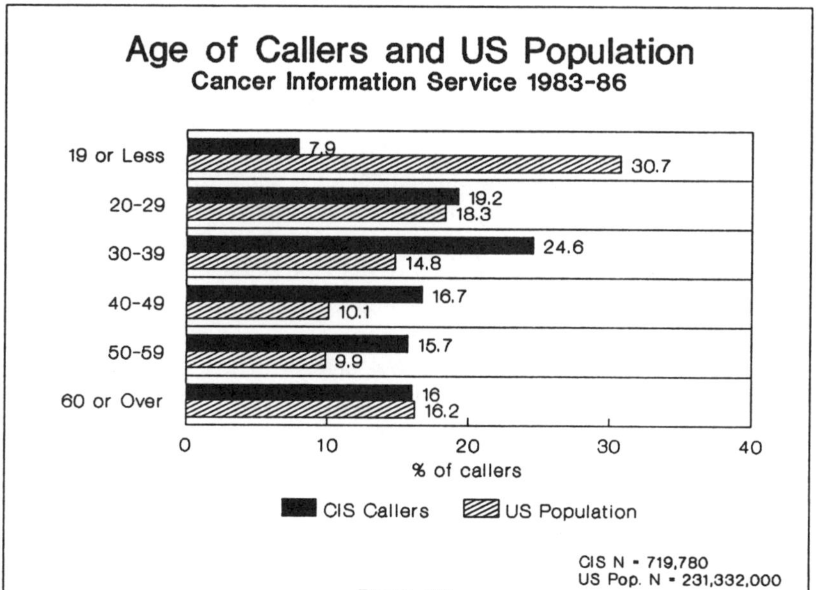

Figure 3.3

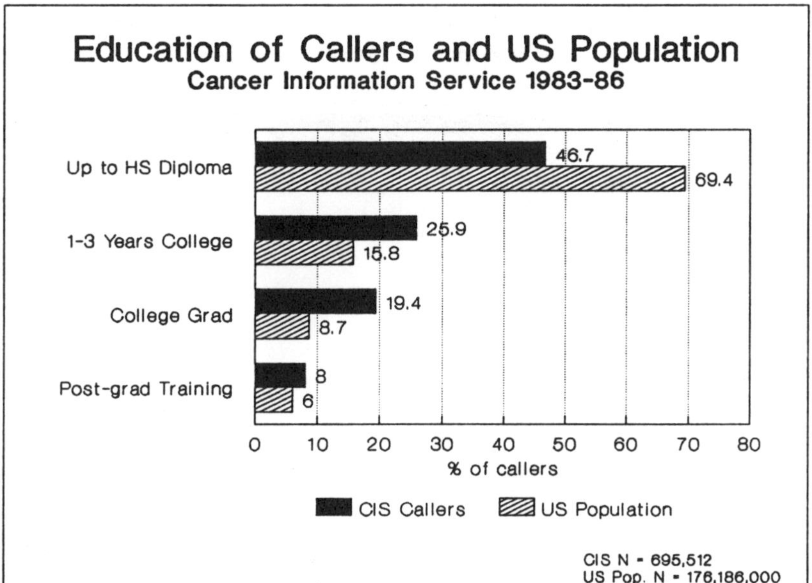

Figure 3.4

the more educated a person, the more likely he or she would be to use the telephone for health information purposes or to seek information in general.

Ethnicity of callers

Figure 3.5 compares the ethnicity of CIS callers with their representation in the U.S. population. This figure illustrates that the CIS is used primarily by whites, with almost 88 percent of CIS users being white compared to their 80 percent share of the U.S. population. Blacks comprise 7.6 percent of CIS users compared to their ll.5 percent share of the population. Hispanics, too, are underrepresented, with 2.7 percent of CIS callers Hispanic compared to 6.4 percent of the U.S. population. Although these figures suggest that the CIS is not reaching all population groups equitably, the reason may be one of socio-economic status (SES) rather than minority status. Efforts to reach minorities have met with varying degrees of success, and in many cases elicit high SES minority callers not unlike white callers demographically; that is, they are a better educated group perhaps more likely to seek health information. These ethnic distributions are discussed more completely in Chapter Nine.

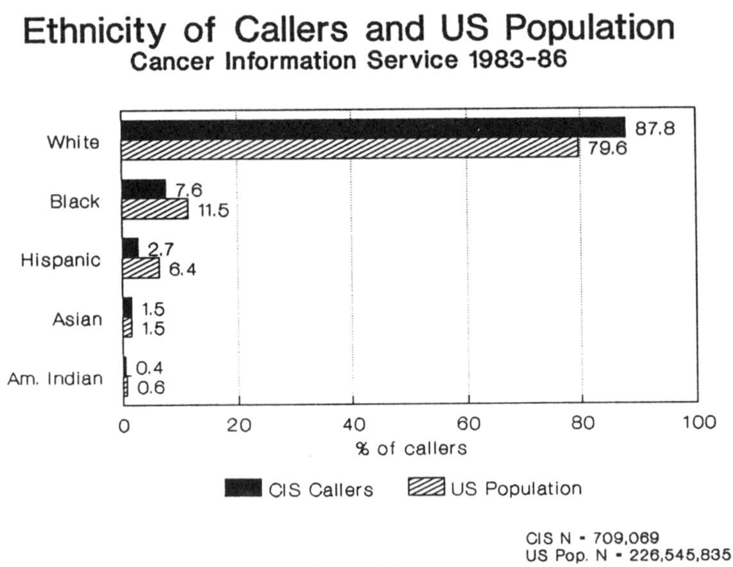

Figure 3.5

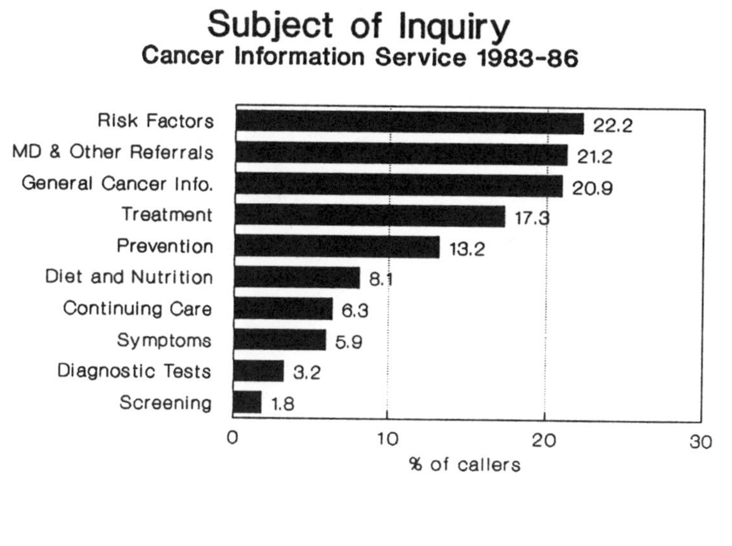

Figure 3.6

What Do Callers Ask About?

Calls are classified according to the subject of their inquiry. For the purpose of this analysis, the original 56 subjects were collapsed into ten general categories. (See Figure 3.6.)

Questions about risk factors

Information on cancer risk factors accounted for over 22 percent of all CIS inquiries, with questions concerning smoking and other tobacco use accounting for over 77 percent of those calls. Typical smoking-related calls concerned information about local smoking cessation programs, requests for "how-to" information on cessation, and requests for advice on how to help others quit smoking. Other risk factors eliciting information requests included exposure to DES, asbestos, radiation, and other occupation and lifestyle risks. Examples of questions asked of the CIS regarding risk factors were:

> "My doctor recommended estrogen for my hot flashes. Will this cause cancer?"

"I work in an office where smoking is allowed. Does this increase my risk of developing lung cancer?"

"Is cancer contagious?"

"Is cancer hereditary? What are my chances of getting it since I have so much in my family?"

"What do you consider 'too many' x-rays?"

"How does chewing tobacco cause cancer?"

"Are tanning booths safe?"

"How can I determine if my mother took DES while she was carrying me?"

"Is it safe to cook food in microwave ovens?"

Questions about referrals

More than 21 percent of inquiries concerned physician referrals or help in accessing community organizations and services, such as the American Cancer Society (ACS), patient support services, financial aid, counseling, cancer detection clinics, and transportation. The large number of inquiries in this category points out the importance of the regional aspect of the program, where these local resources are compiled and maintained in each office. Some examples of questions on physician referrals and local resources include:

"I am having trouble coping with my friend's cancer. Is there anyone I can talk to about this? What resources are available nearby?"

"Is there any financial assistance available for a cancer patient?"

"Where can I go to be tested for the AIDS virus?"

"My doctor says I need surgery. I want a second opinion. Can you give me some doctors' names?"

General cancer questions

Almost 21 percent of inquiries were questions of a general nature, sometimes pertaining to a particular cancer site, and sometimes regarding the overall topic of cancer. This category also includes questions on cancer statistics, and general information about the NCI and research not involving human subjects (human research, or clinical trials, was coded in the treatment category). For example:

> "I am doing a school paper on breast cancer. Can you provide me with information?"
>
> "How many people in my state were diagnosed as having cancer last year?"
>
> "Tell me all you can about colon cancer."
>
> "How does cancer develop and spread?"

Questions about treatment

Inquiries related to cancer treatment accounted for over 17 percent of CIS calls. Often, clarification is sought about treatment options available for a particular type of cancer or the caller is seeking information about a specific medical procedure. In this category, general questions on cancer treatment dominated, with specific questions about chemotherapy, clinical trials, radiotherapy, surgery, hormonal therapy, and immunotherapy accounting for the remainder of the questions. Examples of treatment-related questions included:

> "How does chemotherapy work?"
>
> "I have received the recommended course of treatment for my cancer. The cancer has recurred. How can I participate in clinical trials?"
>
> "What are the alternative treatments for breast cancer?"
>
> "How do I find out what new treatment is available for my type of cancer?"
>
> "Am I receiving the correct treatment for my leukemia?"

Unproven methods for treating cancer, such as laetrile, accounted for almost one percent of these inquiries.

Questions about prevention

Questions on cancer prevention were asked by over 13 percent of CIS users. This category included general questions on cancer prevention and prevention questions on topics other than smoking cessation, such as:

> "What can I do to prevent cancer?"

Questions about diet and nutrition

Diet and nutrition questions comprised over 8 percent of calls and they covered cancer prevention, as well as diet issues related to various cancer treatments. For example:

> "What kind of foods should I eat to reduce my chances of getting cancer?"
>
> "How can I stay as healthy as possible while I am taking chemotherapy treatments?"

Questions about continuing care

Questions on continuing care accounted for over 6 percent of inquiries, including questions related to the doctor-patient relationship; side effects or complications of a particular cancer treatment; pain control; prognosis; and physical or occupational rehabilitation. Some questions in this area were:

> "I have been experiencing swelling in my arm following my mastectomy. Can you tell me what causes this and what I can do?"
>
> "My doctor uses words that I don't understand but I feel awkward asking him to explain them. How can I approach him?"
>
> "I am being discriminated against at work because I have been out for so long following my cancer treatments. How can I deal with my co-workers' insensitivity?"

Questions about symptoms

Just under 6 percent of all inquiries concerned symptoms, with some callers seeking advice about symptoms they suspected as being cancer-related, such as:

> "Is a lump in the breast a sign of breast cancer?"
>
> "I have a mole that has changed color. How do I know if it's cancer?"

Questions about diagnostic procedures

Another 3.2 percent wanted clarification of a particular diagnostic procedure. For example:

> "I am a smoker with respiratory problems. How should I be tested to see if it's cancer?"
>
> "My mammogram is positive. What should I do next?"
>
> "How is a bone scan done?"

Questions about screening

Questions on screening accounted for almost 2 percent of calls and may have been specific to certain cancer types, or general in nature. Questions on this topic include:

> "Can you tell me the elements of a good physical examination for cancer?"
>
> "How much radiation do I get with a routine mammogram?"
>
> "I have a class III Pap smear. What does that mean?"
>
> "Is there a screening test for colon cancer?"

What Cancer Sites Were Asked About?

Forty-one percent of callers asked about a particular cancer site. Figure 3.7 lists the seven sites most commonly inquired about by CIS users. Of these, breast cancer was the most frequent concern, comprising over 26 percent of site-related calls. Cancers of the colon and rectum were of concern to more than 11 percent of those asking about a particular cancer site, and lung cancer by almost that many site-specific callers. The nature of specific questions asked about cancer sites varied greatly from one site to another, and covered the categories of prevention, screening methods, detection tests, treatments, rehabilitation, continuing care, and coping with the disease. Some examples of questions specific to commonly asked-about sites include the following:

> "My mother and aunt died of breast cancer at an early age. Does that increase my risk of getting breast cancer?"
>
> "What is the relationship between cysts in the breast and breast cancer?"
>
> "Can breasts be reconstructed following surgery for breast cancer?"

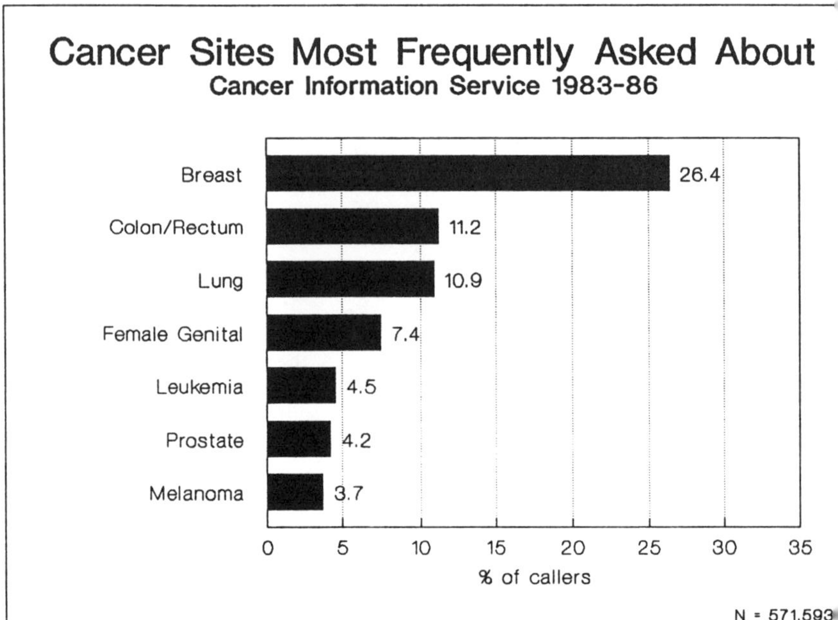

Figure 3.7

"Is lung cancer always fatal?"

"I have lung cancer. Can my small children 'catch it'?"

"What are the symptoms of colon cancer. How is it detected?"

"How can I protect myself from skin cancer when I am in the sun?"

"My menstrual cycle is returning after three years of menopause. Should I worry about cancer?"

"What does a Pap smear reveal?"

Table 3.1 compares the ranking of CIS calls on those sites most commonly inquired about with the estimates of new cancer cases for 1987 (ACS Facts and Figures, 1987). The sites most frequently asked about are somewhat consistent with their incidence in the U.S. population, with the top three cancer sites the same in both lists.

Table 3.1
Rank Comparison CIS Calls/US Cancer Incidence
Cancer Information Service 1983–86

CIS calls	Estimated new cases, 1987
1. Breast	1. Lung
2. Colon/rectum	2. Colon/rectum
3. Lung	3. Breast
4. Female genital	4. Prostate
5. Leukemia	5. Uterus
6. Prostate	6. Bladder
7. Melanoma of skin	7. Oral

How Did Callers Learn of the CIS?

Callers first learned of the CIS through a variety of sources, the majority being media-related, as noted in Figure 3.8. Almost 44 percent of users learned of the CIS through the electronic media. Television was the most common source, having reached more than 39 percent of users. Radio was considerably less important, accounting for only four percent

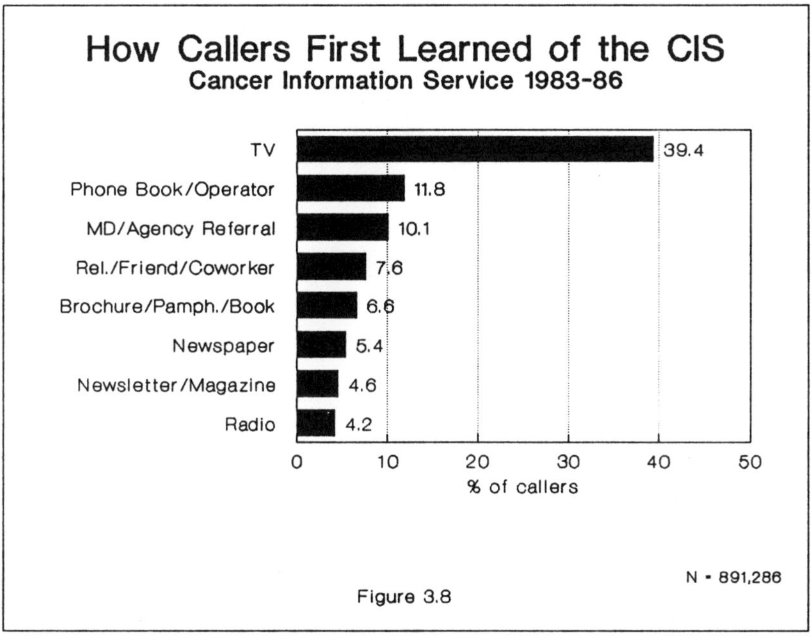

Figure 3.8

of calls. The print media, including newspapers, magazines, pamphlets, brochures, and books accounted for almost 17 percent of inquiries. Almost 12 percent of callers reported they first learned about the CIS by consulting their telephone books or directory assistance. Health professionals, including physicians, and health agencies were responsible for informing more than 10 percent of users about the CIS. Word of mouth, through friends, relatives, neighbors and co-workers, informed almost 8 percent of system users.

Description of Responses to Calls

Behavioral Suggestions

Quite frequently, callers are offered behavioral suggestions for actions to take following their conversation with CIS staff. A total of 906,457 suggestions were offered to callers during the four years, with Table 3.2 illustrating the nature of the suggestions. Almost 39 percent of callers were advised to contact a community agency or service, including the ACS, hospitals and clinics, cancer centers, counseling or support groups, and hospices. Almost 28 percent of callers were directed to talk to or visit their physician or to obtain a second opinion from another physician. In keeping with the concern users displayed about smoking and tobacco use, almost 11 percent of callers were urged to stop or reduce their smoking habit. Approximately the same percent of callers were asked to encourage another person to call the CIS with their concerns. Much smaller numbers of callers were urged to reduce their exposure to particular health hazards, such as x-rays or asbestos, or to learn or practice a self-detection technique, such as breast self-examination or testicular self-examination.

Table 3.2
Behavioral Suggestions for Callers
Cancer Information Service 1983–86

Behavioral suggestions/actions	Callers
Contact other agency/service	38.8%
Talk to or visit physician/second opinion	27.6%
Have another person call CIS	10.9%
Stop/reduce smoking	10.8%
Share information with others	10.2%
Less exposure to health hazards	1.3%
Learn/practice self-detection	1.2%

Time and Follow-Up

CIS staff record the amount of time spent with each inquiry, both on the telephone and after the call. Off-phone time may be spent researching the caller's question, making additional telephone calls to consultants, or gathering information for the caller. On the phone, the majority of inquiries averaged 1—5 minutes in duration (66.7%). Calls lasting 6—15 minutes accounted for 24.3 percent of all inquiries, and calls longer than 15 minutes took up 7.1 percent of the total. Another 1—5 minutes was spent off the telephone on 61.3 percent of the calls, with 30.5 percent requiring no additional time off of the telephone. Staff spent between 6—15 minutes handling 5.4 percent of inquiries and an additional 2.9 percent required over 15 additional minutes of staff time following the telephone contact. Follow-up on the call could involve sending publications (61.7%), calling back with additional information (2.8%), or sending a letter (1.2%). No follow-up was required for 35.1 percent of the calls.

Geographic Distribution of Users

Since the CIS is a "national" program, geographic distribution of users has long been of interest to the various regional offices and the NCI. However, each of the two primary measures of geographical distribution available, total call volume and call rate per 100,000 population have inherent biases. Total call volume favors the offices which have the larger population bases (and usually the largest operating budgets), while call rates per 100,000 population favor those offices with lower population bases in that fewer calls are required to register a particular sized increase or decrease in the call rate.

Figure 3.9 illustrates the number of inquiries to each state during the reporting period (1983—1986). Alaska had the fewest CIS calls, while California had the most. It is important to note that California's calls are divided between two regional offices which share calls from the state's population. The annual call rate during this four-year period for all states combined was 201.44 per 100,000 population. In states where regional offices are located, the annual call rate is 216.3 per 100,000 population; in states where no regional offices is located and the national office handles the calls, the figure drops to 133.5 calls per 100,000 population. These differences between regional and national levels point out one of the benefits of the program's regionalization, where local promo-

Number of CIS Inquiries by State
1983-86

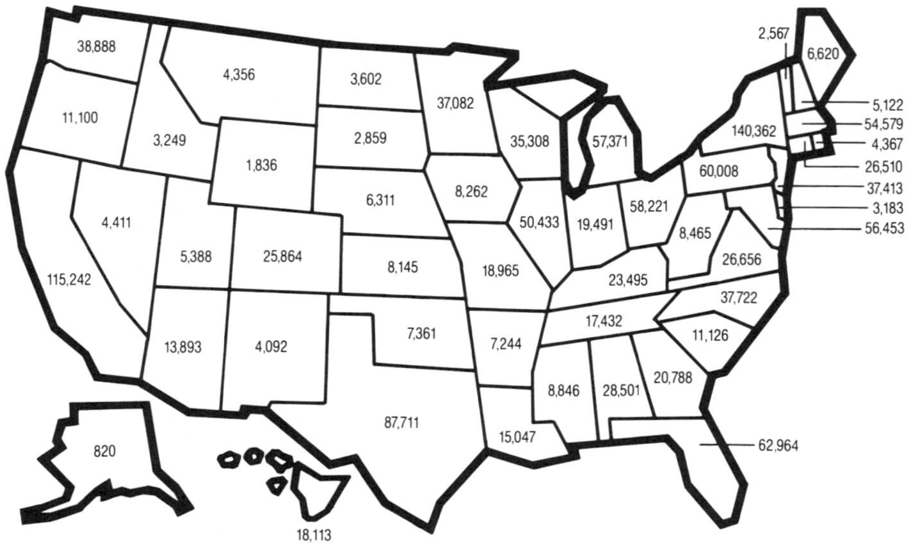

Figure 3.9

tion activities and contacts can increase the proportion of the population served by the CIS.

It should be noted that when computing call rates per 100,000 population, we excluded eight states and the District of Columbia from the calculations. Seven of these states and the District were excluded because they either opened or closed a regional CIS office during the years covered by the study and, thus, were not exclusively in one category or the other for the full time period. Alaska was excluded because it did not have access to the CIS system through the same "800" telephone number as did the rest of the country.

User Survey Response to the CIS

Background and Data Collection Methods

Because the CIS interacts directly with the American public, user satisfaction is of critical importance in determining the value of the program. Equally important are the health-related actions taken following callers' interactions with CIS staff. To assess user satisfaction with CIS and its impact on their health behavior, a mailed survey (see Appendix D) was distributed to a sample of CIS users from January, 1984 through April, 1985. A survey coordinator in each regional office administered the survey locally, and the data were analyzed centrally at NCI. The survey resulted in a response rate of 64.7 percent, with 7,530 questionnaires returned.

Description of the survey instrument

The survey questions were designed to evaluate the following issues:

- The degree to which the CIS is able to meet informational needs of its users;
- The relative effectiveness of the CIS, compared to other information sources, in affecting users' health behavior; and
- The degree to which contact with the CIS influences the health behavior of users.

In order to respond to these issues, callers were asked to specify the reason that they called the CIS, whether they would call again, and if they referred others to the CIS. They were queried on their impressions of CIS staff members and the helpfulness of the information received.

The printed materials mailed to callers and their utility were also evaluated. In order to determine the effectiveness of the CIS in modifying health behavior, callers were asked what their usual sources of information were regarding health issues and how the CIS compared to these other sources in their decision to take a health-related action. Questions regarding referral issues and diffusion of the information received were also included. Finally, a number of administrative questions were asked to identify any difficulties encountered by callers in accessing the CIS office. These questions related to such problems as callers' attempts to locate the CIS telephone number, busy signals, and the length of time the caller was put on "hold."

The user survey was developed through an iterative process involving an Evaluation Task Force with comments from CIS regional office staff. Several different versions of the survey were pilot-tested in four different offices, resulting in a 50 percent response rate with no follow-up. On the basis of the pilot test, the survey instrument and procedures were modified and an operations manual and training program developed.

The survey procedure used by regional offices consisted of several steps during a seven week cycle. Questionnaires were mailed two weeks after the call if a user was selected to participate. Four weeks following the call a post card reminder was sent if a response had not been received. Five weeks from the date of the call a follow-up letter and a second survey form were mailed if no response had yet been received. At the seventh week, no more responses were accepted.

Sampling design

The sample of users who received the survey was derived from all callers who were sent publications or follow-up letters as a result of contact with the CIS and who called on days which were randomly selected for each individual CIS office. Thus the sampling design should have eliminated any systematic bias in the results based on temporal or regional effects (e.g., local staffing patterns). A federal government regulatory office required that the user survey sampling frame consist of only those individuals who received a follow-up mailing of materials as a result of their contact with the CIS. Therefore, the final sampling frame consists of 50.0 percent of all CIS callers on the randomly-sampled days during the survey period.

Sampling days were selected for each regional office such that any one office would receive at least a minimum number of responses sufficient to analyze its individual data locally. The results reported here look at the national data in its aggregate form.

Comparison of respondents with non-respondents

A comparison of the demographic data between respondents and non-respondents to the survey and those not included in the sampling frame because they received no follow-up mailing is presented in Table 3.3. The table first compares CIS users who were part of the survey and other callers on survey days who were not because they received no follow-up materials by mail. There is almost no difference in the two groups based on sex of the caller. While both groups are predominantly white, there were proportionately fewer blacks and more Hispanics and Asians in callers who were surveyed. Educational status in the two groups was very similar. Callers who were surveyed included proportionately more cancer patients and their families and friends and fewer symptomatic users/families/friends and members of the general public. Overall, however, the two groups are proportionately similar in most respects.

Within study subjects, a comparison of respondents and non-respondents yields a similar outcome with slightly more variation than in the previous comparison. There were slightly more males proportionately in the non-respondent group. There are some race/ethnic differences in the two groups, although not widely divergent. Among non-respondents

Table 3.3
User Survey Population Comparisons (in percents)
Cancer Information Service 1984–85

	Non-subjects[a]	Subjects	Respondents	Non-respondents
Male	28.8	28.7	26.9	32.0
Female	71.2	71.3	73.1	68.0
White	84.9	87.8	90.4	83.2
Black	11.1	6.6	5.0	9.6
Hispanic	1.7	2.9	2.5	3.7
Asian	2.1	2.3	1.8	3.3
American Indian	.2	.3	.4	.2
Less than HS	8.8	10.0	8.8	12.2
HS graduate	35.4	32.7	32.2	33.6
Some college	25.6	26.3	27.2	24.7
College grad.	30.2	31.0	31.7	29.5
Patients' family/friends	33.2	39.7	44.4	31.2
Symptomatic family/friends	9.6	8.3	8.5	7.9
General public	56.6	51.7	46.8	60.6

[a]Callers on survey days who were not mailed follow-up materials and thus were not part of the sampling frame.

there are proportionately fewer whites and more blacks, Hispanics, and Asians. Also, among non-respondents there are slightly more individuals with a high school education or less. Only in the types of user comparisons are there somewhat marked differences. Proportionately, there are 13.2 percent more callers in the cancer patients and family/friends category among respondents than non-respondents. The two groups are similar for symptomatic callers and family/friends. There are 13.8 percent more callers from the general public in the non-respondent group than among respondents. It could be speculated that cancer patients see a more immediate need and benefit to their contact with the CIS and are, therefore, more inclined to respond to a survey such as this and thus, be over-represented in the resulting sample.

Overall, for both comparisons the groups are quite similar, except for some differences in ethnic background and type of users. Both of these variable are followed more closely as we analyze the results of the CIS evaluation in more detail throughout the chapters that follow.

Survey Results

User satisfaction

Almost 30 percent of respondents took time to provide handwritten comments elaborating on their interaction with the CIS. Of these, the vast majority were complimentary (90.3% positive, 5.3% neutral, 4.3% negative). Representative comments will be used in this section to illustrate the data obtained from the user survey. In general, survey respondents indicated a high level of satisfaction with CIS in areas of information received, staff and overall usefulness. For example:

> "It is a wonderful service. There are so many questions one can have about cancer, and one doesn't feel free to call a physician for all of them."

> "If I have any questions that are bothering me I will continue to contact CIS and I feel confident they will do what they can to help. I feel they are qualified to do so."

> "Thanking you most sincerely for the prompt service you gave us at this most critical time."

More than 96 percent of the respondents found the information given clear and easy to understand, 94.9 percent found it helpful and 97.6 percent indicated they would call the CIS in the future for answers to other questions about cancer. Almost 50 percent of respondents had already recommended the CIS to others at the time they were surveyed. Respondents found the CIS staff knowledgeable (94.8%), courteous (96.8%) and friendly and sympathetic (96.7%):

> "I really appreciated the time they took to talk to me. I needed someone to listen to me and understand the loss of my mother plus the fear of getting cancer myself."
>
> "Your service is of immeasurable help and comfort when you need to have questions answered. It's nice to have information available and a kind, understanding person to talk to."

Almost 94 percent of the respondents labeled themselves very (78.7%) or somewhat (14.9%) satisfied with their overall use of the CIS, while only 2.1 percent were somewhat or very dissatisfied. In many of these cases, callers' dissatisfaction was the result of not getting the answers they wanted to hear, even though the information offered was correct. For example:

> "I called to find out if the symptoms I had were related to cancer. They told me I should go to see my doctor. I don't like to go to the doctor for every little thing. I will wait and see if it gets worse."

We learned of another source of users' frustration when asking whether or not they had trouble reaching the CIS due to busy signals. Over 16 percent of respondents stated that they received a busy signal when they first called the CIS. This response led to further study of the problem and a number of management decisions to lessen the busy signal rate. These problems and solutions were discussed more fully in Chapter Two. It was gratifying that less than 2 percent of callers felt that they had been put on "hold" for an unreasonable length of time.

When asked what they liked most about the CIS, respondents most often cited the prompt response when they called (79.3%); the "useful" information (78.3%); the courteous and sympathetic staff member (74.1%); the clear and understandable information (74.2%); and the fact that the service was free (69.1%). In responding to what they liked least about the CIS, 66.5 percent responded, "Nothing was unsatisfactory;" busy signals (10.6%); the fact that the telephone number was hard to find

(6.2%); and the fact that a staff member was not immediately available (3.4%) accounted for most of the remaining responses.

Motivation for use of the CIS

Respondents were asked to identify the statement that best described their reason for calling the CIS. The answers most often given were, "I needed an explanation of something I heard (or read) from another source" (32.3%); "I wanted to know if the information I obtained from another source was correct" (30.1%); "I wanted to obtain a pamphlet which was advertised on TV or radio" (37%); and "I wanted to obtain information I could not find elsewhere" (30.6%). Over 9 percent of respondents wanted referrals to a physician, agency or service, and 12 percent simply needed "someone to talk to." These responses point out the public's need for verification of information received from other sources.

Usefulness of information

Respondents were also queried on whether or not the information received was new to them, and 54.2 percent responded affirmatively. Of those calling who received information related to what they already possessed, over 90 percent stated that the information provided by CIS was in agreement with what they already knew before calling, and 77.2 percent agreed that the information provided by CIS was more informative than similar information they had obtained from the other sources.

Diffusion of information

An important issue identified in the user survey was the diffusion of information provided by CIS staff. When questioned about the number of other people the information was shared with, we found that information provided to 4,091 callers reached 11,086 people, almost a three-fold increase. This figure points out the potential for reaching many more people than actually place calls themselves. In fact, to extrapolate this information over a typical year's telephone calls, it could be estimated that information provided to 400,000 CIS users yearly actually reaches 1.1 million people.

Behavioral Response

As important as user satisfaction is the health related action prompted by the contact with CIS. Slightly more than 93 percent of the callers surveyed responded that they had taken some action following their call. The three most common actions taken were reading the materials mailed by the CIS (82.7%), sharing the information with at least one other person (58.4%) and going to or making an appointment with a doctor, clinic or hospital (24.3%). For example:

> "I was very satisfied with the service I received. I used some of the helpful hints in the pamphlet I received and I have quit smoking."
>
> "I was very impressed with the lady I spoke with. She helped me decide to finish my chemo treatments. It also helped me from going from doctor to doctor trying to find the easiest way to continue my treatment."
>
> "This was the best call I made (for information) as a result of my call, the whole family is now being helped. Thank you and God bless you for being there."

Other actions taken following contact with the CIS included seeking more information (18.8%); changing eating habits (16%); attempting to stop or reduce smoking (12%); learning or practicing a self-detection technique (e.g., breast self-examination) (10.4%); reducing environmental exposures such as sunbathing (8.2%); and contacting a community agency or service (5.2%).

Behavioral Influences

The survey acknowledged that sometimes peoples' actions are influenced by many individuals or sources, and asked respondents which of these sources influenced the health actions they had previously described. Relatives and/or friends were most frequently cited as influences on health behavior (42.9%), followed by the mass media, including TV, radio, newspapers and magazines (28.8%). Physicians ranked third as a source of influence, with 19.4 percent of users claiming that their physicians influenced their health behavior described in the survey. Other influences included cancer organizations (11.6%) such as the American Cancer Society, scientific or professional magazines or journals (10.3%), and other health professionals (8.1%), such as a nurse or a pharmacist. Almost 14 percent of users reported that none of the listed sources influenced their health behavior in this instance.

When asked about the relative importance of their contact with the CIS in their decision to take health-related action, almost 92 percent of callers said that their contact with the CIS was very (57.6%) or somewhat

(33.9%) important. Another 5.4 percent said contact with the CIS was not very important, and 3.2 percent said it was not important at all.

Summary

The CIS evaluation design consists of three parts: a call record form (CRF) completed on every inquiry to the CIS, a user survey, and a quality control assessment. The first two of these elements are discussed in this chapter.

The CRF collects three types of information: administrative (e.g., date, location, time); inquiry/response (e.g., caller type, subject of inquiry, and site); and user demographics (e.g., age, education, sex). As part of a pilot test of the CRF, an analysis of inter-coder agreement demonstrated reasonable levels of agreement even on complex multi-coded calls.

Results of almost 1.4 million CRFs collected between January, 1983 and December, 1986 showed that almost all inquiries were telephone calls, with over 80 percent being first time CIS users. The most frequent users were members of the general public, followed by family and friends of patients, health professionals, cancer patients, and symptomatic persons and their family and friends. Almost 40 percent of callers asked about a particular cancer site with breast cancer as the most frequent concern, followed by colon/rectum, and lung. In general, sites inquired about more frequently also have the highest incidence in the U.S. population.

The original 56 subject of inquiry codes were collapsed into ten. Almost one-fourth of the callers asked about cancer risk factors, followed by questions about local services, then general cancer information and treatment. The analysis of the demographics revealed that almost three times as many females as males use the CIS. CIS callers tend to be older and better educated than the overall population. The CIS is used primarily by whites. The other ethnic groups are underrepresented among CIS users.

The most prevalent behavioral suggestion given to callers was to contact other local resources as well as their own physicians. According to these results, most CIS users first learned of the service through the media, particularly television. The telephone book also emerged as an important source.

The geographical analysis of callers revealed that states with regional offices had an annual call rate per 100,000 of 216.3 compared to an annual call rate of only 133.5 per 100,000 for those states with no regional office serving their area.

User satisfaction was assessed with a mailed survey sent to a random sample of callers who were sent other mailings. Of those contacted, 64.7 percent responded resulting in over 7,500 questionnaires. Generally, users reported high levels of satisfaction. About half of the respondents had already recommended the service to others. Over half reported that the information from the CIS was new to them and over 90 percent rated their contact with the CIS as very or somewhat important to their subsequent health actions. One problem identified was the difficulty reaching some CIS offices due to busy signals. These survey results indicate that the CIS is perceived as providing a significant service to its users, and is instrumental in helping callers take health related action. Perhaps this caller summed up the CIS best:

> "It's just a darn good information service to have when you need friendly help."

4

Differences Among CIS User Groups

The general results discussed in the previous chapter mask some important differences among the three groups of consumers who use the CIS—the general public, symptomatic people, and cancer patients and their family/friends. (See Appendix E for selected CIS data tables.) In this chapter, we will highlight some of the major differences among these users and in the following chapters we will analyze each of these user groups in more detail.

Caller Demographic Characteristics

The only demographic characteristic which differs substantially among user groups is ethnicity. Figure 4.1 shows the comparison among the ethnic distributions of these three groups. The three ethnic groups analyzed have quite similar distributions across user groups, i.e., most calls are placed by the general public followed by family/friends of patients, patients, and symptomatic individuals.

Proportionately more black and Hispanic than white callers are members of the general public. It may be that the minority groups, because they watch more television, are particularly responsive to PSA campaigns that encourage calling to order free materials. Proportionately more whites are classified as family/friends of cancer patients than are blacks (12%) and Hispanics (17%). Perhaps seeking health information is a more acceptable form of social support among whites than blacks. Proportionately more black callers are symptomatic, both those who have seen and have not seen a doctor, than are whites and Hispanics. This finding could result from the crisis-oriented health care often found in the black community. Blacks may prefer calling a free service to get information on a symptom rather than visiting a health care facility where they may face long waits and compete with much more seriously ill patients.

Ethnicity of User Groups
Cancer Information Service 1983-86

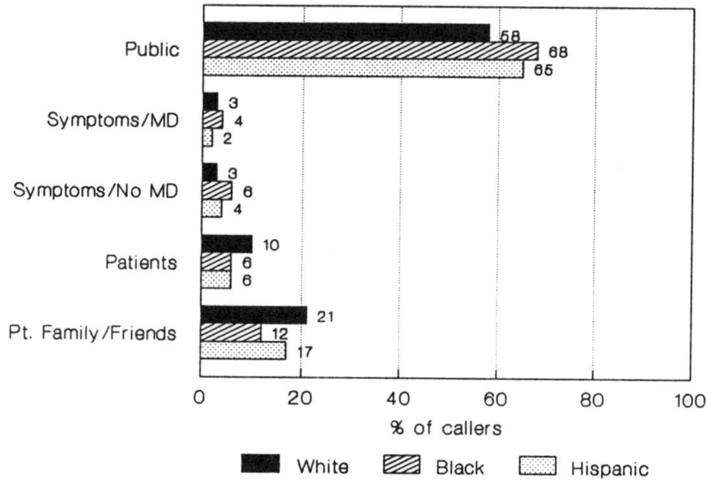

Figure 4.1

% of User Groups That Are Repeat Callers
Cancer Information Service 1983-86

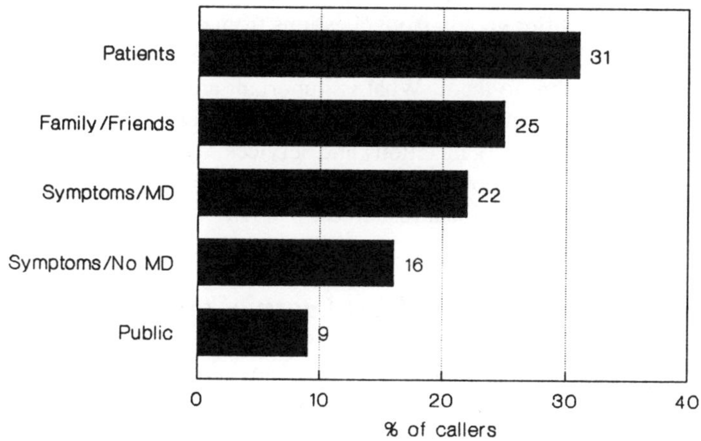

Figure 4.2

Figure 4.2 shows the percentage of the different user groups who have called the CIS before. These results validate the usefulness of the system. As the users move along the disease continuum and become more involved with cancer, the likelihood that they have used the system before increases. Only nine percent of the general public have called the CIS before but 31 percent of the cancer patients have called previously.

What Do the Callers Ask About?

Figure 4.3 focuses on four of the more frequent subjects of inquiry. The different user groups vary dramatically on these subjects of inquiry. The general public are most interested in prevention, particularly smoking and other risk factors; this topic is asked about infrequently by the other three user groups. For symptomatic callers, symptoms are the subject of most interest but there is a difference between those who have seen a doctor and those who have not. Those who have not seen a doctor are more likely to ask about symptoms and less likely to ask about treatment than those who have seen a doctor. Apparently those who have not seen a doctor are at a more preliminary stage of information seeking. They are most interested in the immediate symptoms they are experiencing. On the other hand, those who have seen a doctor are beyond interest in the symptom and more concerned about next steps in the process such as diagnostic tests and treatment.

The subjects cancer patients and family/friends of cancer patients ask about differ greatly from questions from other groups of callers. They have a diagnosed cancer, so risk factors, prevention, and screening are less important to them. What is important are treatment issues and local organizations and services. In fact, all the user groups appear to have an interest in local organizations and services, again validating the need for regional information offices that can collect and maintain up to date information on such local resources.

How Do the Callers First Learn of the CIS?

Figure 4.4 shows that television is an important source of awareness about the CIS for all the user groups but particularly for the general public. Symptomatic people, on the other hand, tend to rely almost equally on the television and the telephone book. Cancer patients and their family/friends show the most heterogeneity for these sources. They report less dependence on television and more on interpersonal sources.

Selected Subject of Inquiry for Different User Groups

Cancer Information Service 1983-86

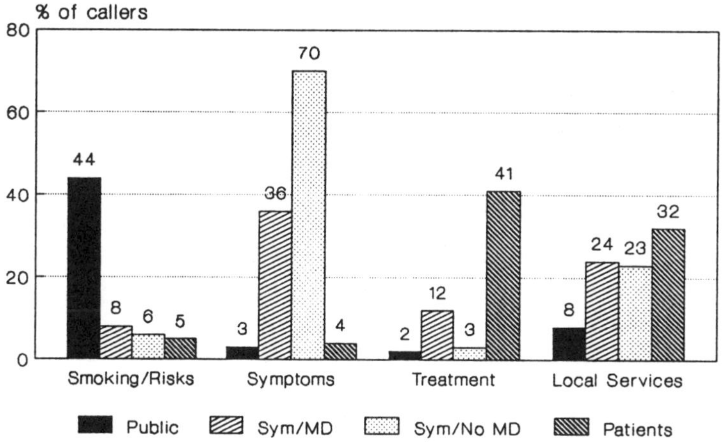

Figure 4.3

How Different User Groups First Learned of the CIS

1983-86

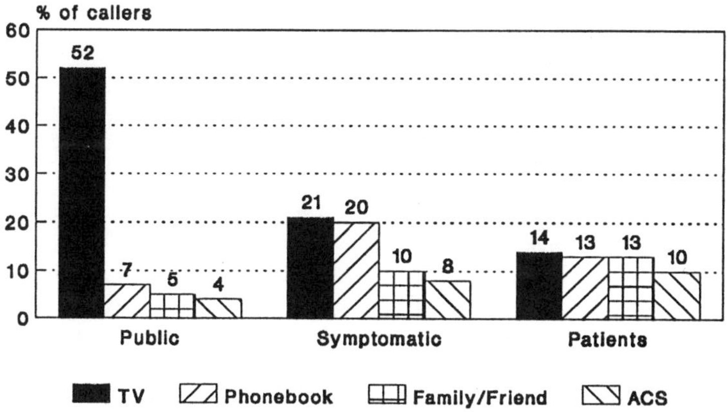

Figure 4.4

How Did the Callers Evaluate the CIS?

Figure 4.5 shows that all groups were highly satisfied with their CIS experience but that symptomatic callers reported the highest satisfaction. Perhaps the reason for the high satisfaction is the positive correlation between satisfaction and having one's "most important question answered by the CIS." Almost 88 percent of the symptomatic callers affirmed that this question was answered—a percentage exceeding those of the other user groups.

Figure 4.6 displays the results of asking how important the CIS call was in influencing subsequent behavioral change. More than half of all the user groups rated the CIS as very important. As might be expected, more symptomatic (63.8%) and patient-related (62.2%) callers rated the CIS as very important than did the general public (51.5%).

The final comparison shown in Figure 4.7 highlights three of ten possible influences for behavioral change which callers were asked to rate. The general public rated the mass media as most influential on their behavioral change. In fact, they were the only user group for whom indirect contact was more influential in behavior change than direct, per-

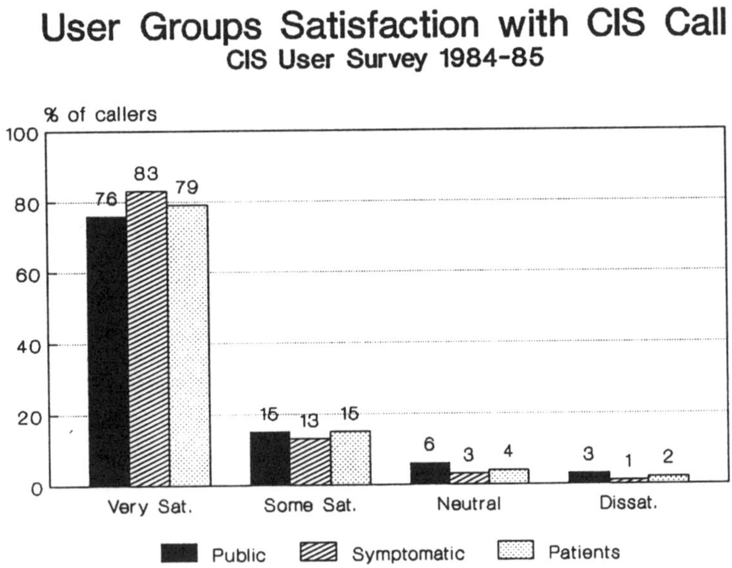

Figure 4.5

Importance of CIS Call in Influencing Behavior

CIS User Survey 1984-85

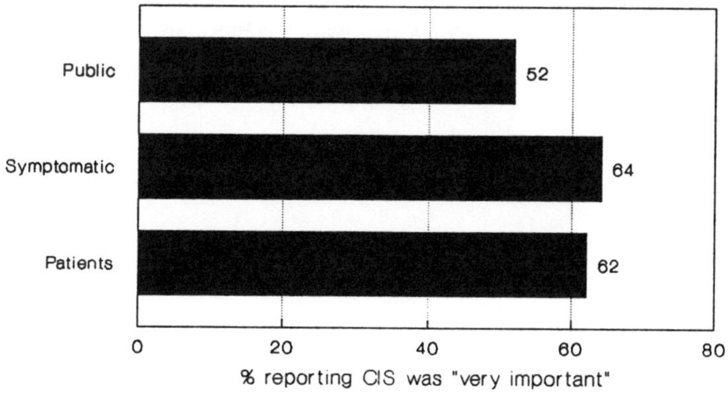

Figure 4.6

Other Influences for Behavior Change

CIS User Survey 1984-85

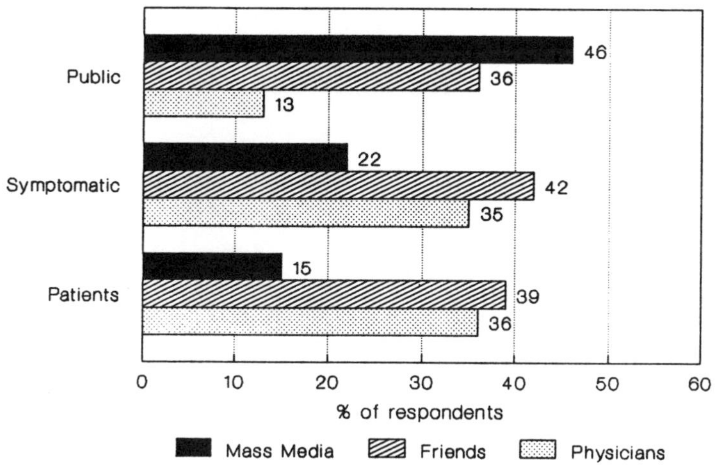

Figure 4.7

sonal contact. Interpersonal contacts including friends and physicians were clearly more important for symptomatic and patient callers.

Chapters Five through Seven each focus on one of the three main CIS user groups defined by their position along the disease continuum. In each chapter, we review the available literature on that group's search for cancer information and present the major findings from the CIS call record form and user survey data bases.

5

The General Public's Search for Cancer Information

We begin with an examination of the general public's search for cancer information because everyone, regardless of his/her eventual experience with cancer, is influenced by previous exposure to the disease as a member of the general public. This previous exposure to information about the disease is part of the individual's underlying beliefs through which current information is interpreted.

Based on our model of the information acquisition process, we would expect the general public to be a much more passive audience for cancer information than are cancer patients and symptomatic persons. We would predict that most stimuli provoking information searches would reach the public incidentally during the course of exposure to mass media and interpersonal communication. We also would expect this group to engage in quite limited information searches and to be primarily interested in those subjects most salient to them, namely cancer prevention and risk factors.

Because of the passive nature of the general public's information seeking little previous research addresses the seeking behaviors directly. Instead, research focuses on the extent of cancer knowledge among the general public. The following sections will describe the limited research on the general public's information seeking behavior plus the more extensive body of literature on the public's knowledge about cancer causes, prevention, detection, and treatment.

The Public's Cancer Information Seeking Behavior

The NCI and the Food and Drug Administration conducted two waves of a telephone survey to assess the public's knowledge, attitudes, and practices related to cancer prevention and risk. The first wave with 1,876 respondents was conducted in June, 1983, prior to beginning a new Cancer Prevention Awareness program. Wave II of the survey was conducted from February to April 1985 during NCI's Cancer Prevention Awareness Campaign and used 1,898 interviews.

Nearly one-half of all respondents in Wave II said they had heard or read about cancer prevention in the preceding six months. They reported that they most frequently used television, newspapers, and magazines as sources of cancer prevention information. The organization or person that most respondents said they would contact for information about cancer prevention was the American Cancer Society (ACS) (41%), followed by their family doctor (34%). No other potential information source was named by more than three percent of the respondents, and less than one percent mentioned the CIS. In fact, the ACS (95%) was the most widely recognized of the four cancer-related organizations listed, far ahead of NCI (59%), CIS (24%), and the fictitious Williams Cancer Center (6%). Almost 20 percent of respondents in Wave II said they had heard of NCI's toll-free number for cancer information (1-800-4-CANCER), and three percent had actually called the number.

Public's Level of Cancer Knowledge

Most of the resources used in this description were surveys identified and summarized by National Analysts (Division of Booz-Allen and Hamilton Inc.) for the National Cancer Institute as the first phase of the National Survey of Public Knowledge, Attitudes and Practices Relating to Cancer. In addition, National Analysts conducted 16 group depth interviews with members of the general public and key subgroups in January and February, 1982. Group depth interviews are a qualitative research method designed to be exploratory rather than definitive. Data from these group interviews are not based on random samples and are not statistically projectable to the broader population.

Respondents in group depth interviews were able to give the following fragmented words or phrases as their understanding of cancer: virus, infection, germs, uncontrollable growth of cells, abnormal growths, deterioration of cells, and sores (National Analysts, 1982). In general, the public underestimate the incidence of cancer in the population but overestimate cancer mortality. Personal interviews with 1,553 individuals in 1978 (Lieberman, 1979) revealed that the public believe that only one out of seven people will develop cancer in their lifetime. The actual figure is currently one out of three. Moreover, the average estimate of survival from the same survey was one in five while the actual survival rate is one in two. These errors may contribute to an apathy about preventing cancer. If an individual believes that cancer is not that prevalent, it is easier to rationalize that he/she will not get it. On the other hand, if one believes that cancer is almost always fatal, then experiencing a warning signal will lead to feelings of doom, further excusing the individual from any constructive action.

The public seem to know the body sites where cancer most often occurs. The sites most frequently mentioned in the 1980 survey were lung, breast, and skin. One of the most prevalent cancer sites, the colon and rectum, was mentioned by only 36 percent of the respondents (Lieberman, 1979). This percentage probably has increased as a result of the publicity surrounding President Reagan's colon cancer in 1985. Some of the beliefs about cancer which persist in the general public include the following (with clarifying information noted in parenthesis):

1. Cancer is hereditary. (Although most cancers are not "hereditary," family history is a major risk factor for breast cancer, for some melanomas, and for colon/rectum cancer.)
2. Bruises cause cancer. (There is no evidence that bruises cause cancer.)
3. There is more cancer now.
4. Surgery spreads cancer. (A surgical procedure to remove cancerous growth may sometimes result in the spread of cancer.)
5. Cancer is contagious. (There is no evidence that cancer is contagious.) (National Analysts, 1982, pp. 77–78)

Causes of Cancer

When asked about the causes of cancer, the public respond with four broad categories of causes: environment, the food supply, stress, and unknown interaction triggers (medications which either singly or in combination with other medications could trigger cancer). Only 38 percent of Wave II respondents in the NCI/FDA survey believed that cancer is usually caused by people's lifestyles, whereas more than twice that percentage of respondents believed that ulcers (88%) and high blood pressure (77%) were related to lifestyle (NCI, Cancer Prevention Awareness Survey, 1986).

When discussing the environment as a cause of cancer, "cancer is everywhere" was a pervasive undercurrent. All respondents in the group depth interviews (National Analysts, 1982) were aware of x-rays, radiation, and cigarette smoking as environmental pollutants.

The food supply as a potential cause of cancer was of greater concern to women than to men, and of greater concern than epidemiologic evidence supports. Use of artificial ingredients was an important issue to these women.

Although the group depth interviewees did not believe that stress causes cancer per se, they did believe that stress can weaken defenses and make one more susceptible to cancer (National Analysts, 1982).

Even though there is no apparent awareness that tobacco use overshadows all other causes of cancer, a large majority of smokers and nonsmokers believe that a major cause of cancer is smoking. But seven out of ten smokers believe that lung cancer can be cured. (Lieberman, 1978). Actually, lung cancer is one of least curable forms of cancer. Primary prevention through smoking prevention and cessation is the major means of reducing lung cancer.

Cancer Prevention and Detection

The dominant impression one gets from the cancer surveys and group depth report is one of helplessness. Most people seem to believe that there is little they can do to prevent cancer. In fact, in Wave II of the Cancer Prevention Awareness Survey, about half the respondents agreed with the statements, "It seems like everything causes cancer," and "There is not much a person can do to prevent cancer." (NCI, Cancer Prevention Awareness Survey, 1986, p. iv).

Knowledge of cancer's standard warning signals is sparse. Virtually all respondents could correctly identify *unaided* at least one warning signal; nearly none could name the standard seven. Lieberman (1978) reported that the proportion of people able to identify the standard seven warning signals based on *aided* recall ranged from 46 percent for the signals, persistent indigestion and difficulty swallowing, to 85 percent for a lump or thickening in the breast or elsewhere. Some of the group depth interviewees saw detection as useless because in their minds early detection does not make a difference. Many of the lower income respondents rejected detection examinations because of the costs (National Analysts, 1982). Moreover, there is a segment of the public that simply has no knowledge of these detection techniques (National Analysts, 1982). Pap tests and breast self-examination are the two detection techniques which have the highest levels of awareness and practice. Only one in four respondents were aware of the hemoccult test or the stool Guiac test. Nearly half (48%) had heard of the proctoscopic examination and 62 percent were aware of the digital rectal examination.

Treatment

The public can easily identify the conventional cancer treatments: surgery, radiation, and chemotherapy. None of these treatments is viewed as optimal, however. In fact, the conclusion expressed in every group interview was that "treatment is worse than the disease." (National Analysts, 1982). Lieberman (1982) reported that surgery was viewed as more effective, less likely to have side effects, but more painful, than chemotherapy and radiation. The dominant image in the public's mind is that "once a person is diagnosed as having cancer, the prognosis is death preceded by painful, disfiguring treatment." (National Analysts, 1982, p. 75).

Another study (Stone and Seigel, 1986) combined information on prevention, causation, detection, and treatment into one general cancer knowledge level score and examined demographic, behavioral, and attitudinal variables for a sample personally interviewed in Los Angeles. The results showed that nonsmoker as well as ex-smoker status, education, cancer worry, and the number of things done to improve one's health were positively related to cancer knowledge. Hispanic ethnicity, age, black ethnicity, and household size were negatively associated with cancer knowledge. Finally, moderate frequency of health worry predicted more accurate knowledge about cancer than frequent and infrequent health worry. Unfortunately, all these variables explained only 17.5 percent of the variance in cancer knowledge.

In summary, the public are relatively well-informed about cancer, although many misconceptions still prevail. The pessimistic and fatalistic attitudes held about this disease appear to be changing, but only slowly. In the following sections of this chapter, we will examine the general public's information seeking from the Cancer Information Service.

CIS Calls from the General Public

Who are the Callers?

The general public callers include all those callers who are not cancer patients, people with symptoms, families and friends of these two groups, and health professionals. This general public group is the largest of the three types of users we will be discussing, accounting for 46.6 percent of all calls to the CIS between 1983 and 1986. Many of the calls made by the general public were simple requests to order literature they had seen promoted in the mass media.

Of all the user groups we are examining, it is the general public that we would expect to resemble most closely the total U.S. population. Even in this group of callers, women callers (66.5%) outnumber male callers (33.5%) by almost two to one. The general public who call the CIS are more educated than the U.S. population. Half of these callers have at least some college, compared to 30.5 percent of the total population. The general public callers are younger than other CIS callers but still older than the U.S. population. Almost half (45.5%) of the general public callers are between 20 and 40 years old while one-third of the U.S. population falls into these age ranges.

Minorities are underrepresented in the general public calls to the CIS. Figure 5.1 compares the representation of ethnic groups in CIS general public calls and the U.S. population. The problem of stimulating calls from minority groups is exacerbated by their overrepresentation

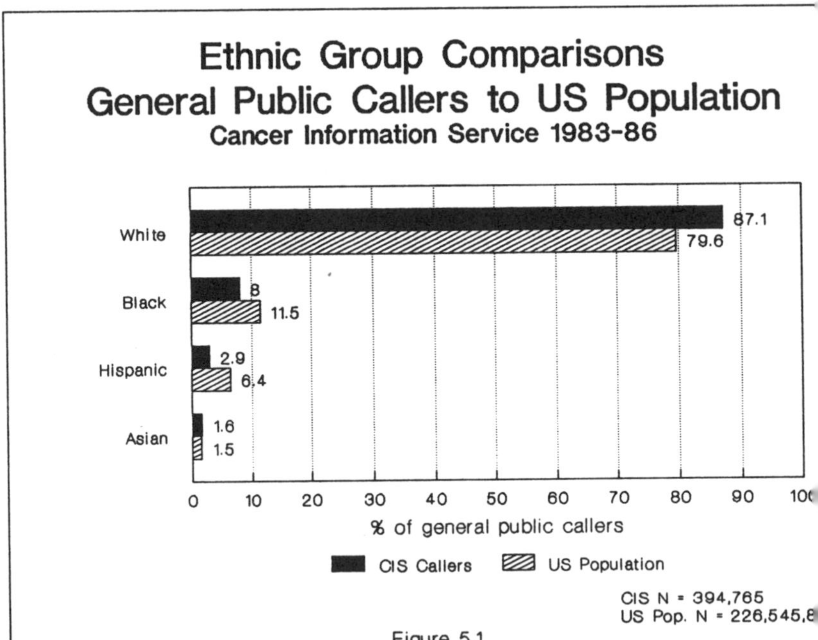

Figure 5.1

among those with low socioeconomic status who traditionally are not active information seekers. This "knowledge gap" phenomenon will be discussed further in Chapter Nine.

What Do These Callers Ask About?

As might be expected, the general public callers are calling to find out how to prevent cancer. Almost half (43.7%) of their questions concern smoking and other risk factors. For example, a male in his twenties who had quit smoking called to ask about his unexplained "side effects." An elderly women asked the CIS where she could get "nicotine gum." Not all of these smoking inquiries are from smokers wanting to quit or ex-smokers. Non-smokers call about their involuntary passive smoking. One white female in her thirties called to ask about the legal rulings governing smoking in the workplace. Another caller, a teenager, asked how she could help her good friend stop smoking. Many of these callers are concerned about presumed cancer risks, such as "aflatoxin in peanut butter," "deodorants," "dry cleaning fluids," "hairdyes," "rays from the TV," "saccharin," and "flying in an airplane because of radiation up in the air."

The second most frequent subject inquired about is general prevention, followed by general cancer information and diet and nutrition. Some examples of diet and nutrition questions include a woman in her sixties who claimed she saw a PSA that said vegetables *cause* cancer, or the man who heard a report on CNN which prompted him to ask about beer consumption and cancer risk. Calls about these topics may have been stimulated by several smoking and cancer prevention media campaigns which will be discussed in Chapter Eight. Men ask about smoking and other risk factors more often than women. In the population at large, not only is the smoking rate higher for men but there is evidence that the quitting rate is higher for men than it is for women. Therefore, one area in which men may be more susceptible to messages encouraging them to utilize the CIS is to get help in "kicking the habit."

The differences in information sought by educational levels occur for the two extreme groups—those with less than high school diplomas and those who are college graduates. The most highly educated callers are more interested in diet and nutrition and prevention but less interested in smoking and other risk factors. This relationship between calls about smoking and education is consistent with smoking rates which are lower for the most educated segments of the population.

Several interesting patterns for age and subject of inquiry were identified. Questions on general prevention, diet and nutrition, local organizations and services and physician referral increased as age increased. It is likely that the threat of cancer becomes more salient as a person gets older and his/her interest in the topic intensifies. Questions about smoking and other risk factors are most frequent for callers 29 or younger and decrease sharply after age 50. Perhaps older people are more likely to have already stopped smoking or have tried to stop unsuccessfully and are resigned to their current habits.

An examination of the nature of the questions for different ethnic groups reveals some interesting differences for Asians. They are much more likely to ask about prevention. Over half of their calls concern this topic versus about a third of the calls from other ethnic groups. In addition, Asians are two to three times more likely to ask about diet and nutrition than the other ethnic groups. Perhaps these questions reflect Asian cultural beliefs about maintaining a healthy balance in their lives.

American Indians ask more often about smoking and other risk factors than do the other ethnic groups, probably reflecting their high smoking rates and use of smokeless tobacco. The only subject that Hispanics ask proportionately more often about is general cancer information.

What Cancer Sites Were Asked About?

Breast (37.7%) is the site most frequently asked about by the general public followed by colon/rectum (19.6%), lung (14.9%), other skin (7.7%), and leukemia (6.4%). Except for leukemia, this list is not surprising, because these are the cancers which are most prevalent and discussed most frequently in the media. Leukemia may be one of the top five sites inquired about because the progress in treating childhood leukemia has received so much media attention. Moreover, childhood leukemia is an emotionally charged experience for all those who know the child, and may prompt more information seeking than other cancers.

As we would expect women asked more often about breast, cervical, and uterine cancer than men. The sites men asked about more frequently were less predictable: colon/rectum, lung, prostate, and melanoma of the skin. The frequency of the questions about prostate cancer from males makes sense since it is a site only affecting males. Calls asking about lung cancer may occur more frequently from males because smoking rates among males are higher. The reasons for the higher proportion of calls from males about colon/rectum cancer is less clear since the incidence for this cancer is similar for males and females. However, the data analyzed here do include the time period that President Reagan's colon cancer received so much media attention. Perhaps this publicity stimulated increased information seeking in many men who identified with the president's problem. There is more uncertainty concerning the higher proportion of questions about melanoma of the skin from male callers.

Education's impact on site inquiries was most pronounced for the number of inquiries about lung cancer by the lowest educated group. Almost one-third of the callers from the group with less than a high school education asked about lung cancer, almost three times as many inquiries as any other education group. This trend is consistent with smoking patterns where the smoking rate is the highest for the less educated groups.

This same group with little education also was two times more likely to call about non-melanoma skin cancer than the other education groups. The less educated group asked less frequently than the other groups about breast, colon/rectum, and cervical cancer.

The trends for age resemble those for education. The under 19 age category asked more frequently about lung, leukemia, and non-melanoma skin cancers. Perhaps lung and other skin cancer are more salient because of the high incidence of smoking and sunbathing in this age group. Leukemia may be more salient because it has an image of a "young person's cancer." Colon/rectum and prostate were two cancers where frequency of questions increased steadily with age.

Table 5.1 illustrates how ethnicity affects the sites inquired about. Some of these results are consistent with incidence data. For example, blacks have more cervical cancer and less skin cancer than other ethnic groups. American Indians smoke and/or use smokeless tobacco more than other ethnic groups, perhaps increasing their interest in lung cancer. Moreover, Hispanics have more cervical cancer. It is less understandable

Table 5.1
Relative Frequency of Site Questions by Ethnicity

Blacks	Hispanics
More cervix Less skin	More cervix More breast
Asians	**American Indians**
Less cervix More skin	Less breast More skin More lung

why Hispanics ask more about breast cancer since their incidence rates are not so high although perhaps their concern is especially intense. It is also less clear why Asians ask more about non-melanoma skin cancers.

How Did the Callers Learn of the CIS?

The public relies heavily on the general mass media to learn about the CIS. The most frequently reported source is television with over one-half of all these callers reporting this source. This reliance on TV is not surprising since much CIS promotion targeted to the general public uses this channel. For example, one young man in his twenties from Beverly Hills called in response to a special program on television about colon cancer, which he said frightened him because he had had "rectal bleeding and terrible diet habits." The telephone book/directory assistance is reported by 8.3 percent, followed by radio (7.9%) and newspapers (6.9%).

There is a gender difference which is consistent with the traditional role of women as information gatherers. Men report greater use of the more passive channels—TV and radio—while women report greater use of the more active sources such as the telephone book, the newspaper, the American Cancer Society, and a newsletter or magazine.

The education of the caller does seem to affect the way he/she first learned of the CIS. The less educated the caller, the more likely that TV is the source reported. On the other hand, the more educated the caller, the greater the likelihood that radio, newspapers, newsletters and magazines, and the American Cancer Society are reported as information sources.

TV as a source of information about the CIS decreases with age while radio and newspapers increase with age. The youngest callers report first learning of the CIS from friends, neighbors, and co-workers more often than the other age groups.

The largest difference among ethnic groups was in their reporting of TV as the source of first information about the CIS. More blacks, Hispanics, and American Indians reported TV than did whites or Asians; the latter were only half as likely to use TV as most other minority groups. Asians relied most heavily on newspapers for information about the CIS, with about 37 percent of all Asians reporting newspapers as their source of information on the CIS compared to between four and seven percent of all other ethnic groups. In fact, 10 percent of all callers reporting newspapers as their source of information about the CIS were Asians, while Asians comprise only about 1.6 percent of all callers. Clearly, this group is responsive to the written word.

Description of Responses to Calls

Behavioral Suggestions

Almost two-thirds (63.2%) of these general public callers were advised to read literature being sent to them and about one-fourth were counseled to attempt to stop or reduce smoking. More males than females were advised to stop smoking.

Fewer college graduates were told to try to quit smoking, but this difference probably only reflects the lower frequency of calls about smoking from this well-educated group. The least educated group were twice as likely to be told to share information obtained with others. Since this same pattern appears with the age 19 or younger callers, perhaps this group contains many young people who were asked to share information with their parents or friends.

The suggestion to stop smoking peaks for callers age 20–29 (36.6%) and then decreases with age (11% by age 60 and over). Perhaps more younger people are communicating an interest in quitting or the information specialists on the phones are assuming that it is easier to change behavior at younger ages and are therefore more likely to suggest modifications of smoking habits to younger people.

Ethnicity did appear to have isolated effects on behavioral suggestions made to callers. American Indians were more frequently advised to quit smoking. Hispanics were more likely to be told to reduce their exposure to occupational health hazards. The most interesting pattern involved Asians, who were more frequently referred to physicians, the American Cancer Society, hospitals and clinics, and cancer centers. The Asian callers may be particularly assertive information seekers who are perhaps less likely to settle for advice such as reading the literature, and hence probed for more specific suggestions.

Time on the Phone

In general, calls from the general public are handled quickly—87.9 percent taking less than five minutes. There were no significant relationships between demographic groups and time spent on the phone.

Follow-Up to the Phone Inquiry

Over three-fourths of the callers from the general public received publications as a follow-up. Gender, education and age did not seem to affect the nature of the follow-up. Ethnicity, however, did seem to affect the follow-up. Hispanics were more likely to be sent publications and to be called back.

About 80 percent of the calls which required follow-up could be handled in less than five minutes. Less than four percent required more than six minutes.

User Response to the CIS

User Satisfaction

On a five-option Likert scale ranging from "very satisfied" to "very dissatisfied," 75.9 percent of the general public were "very satisfied" with the CIS. One general public caller from Florida expressed his satisfaction in the following way:

> Thank you all (for) sending any and all information that might relate, by hearing what is said, and not said, you have convinced me. Evidence, facts and figures did it and you all provided them to me. I am so very gratful (sic.) for this service. Have told various of my co-workers about it. For myself, I broke my pipes in two. In no way will I ever insult my lungs again by smoking. This can be attributed to you all being on the other end of the line and with the facts.

In all, satisfaction was expressed by 91.3 percent of the general public callers, 6.2 percent were "neither satisfied nor dissatisfied," and the remaining 2.5 percent were dissatisfied with the CIS. Levels of dissatisfaction may depend partly on receipt of the materials requested. One dissatisfied caller complained:

> After 17 years of smoking, I need to stop and want to cooperate with my doctor in getting my health back. I'm frustrated by your lack of response. It's been two weeks since I asked for the information.

Behavioral Response

The only behaviors with which the general public did not comply to an extent similar to that suggested by the CIS were referrals. About 10.8 percent of the callers were referred to clinics, physicians, hospitals, agen-

Table 5.2
Comparison of Behavioral Suggestions with Actions Taken
General Public Callers (user survey respondents)

Behavioral suggestions/actions	Percent told	Percent did
Read materials sent	77.3	81.3
Stop/reduce smoking	12.6	18.7
Share information with others	10.4	50.6
Referred agency/service	8.2	2.5
See personal physician	7.3	7.5
Reduce exposure to environmental health hazards	4.7	12.0
Learn self-detection techniques	3.4	12.2
Referred clinic/physician/hospital	2.6	1.5
Seek second opinion	.7	2.2
Change eating habits	—[a]	21.2

[a]Although 21.2 percent reported a change in eating habits, this category is not specifically listed under behavioral suggestions on the CRF.

cies and/or services, but only 4 percent followed through by contacting or visiting the referral.

When evaluating the success of behavioral change or action, it is useful to review the reason(s) for the calls. Almost two-thirds of the general public callers (63.8%) said that their main reason for calling was to request literature which was advertised on television. One respondent wrote: "I wanted information that I could understand and refer back to."

Of those receiving literature, 81.3 percent recorded that they read the materials sent to them. Table 5.2 shows a comparative breakdown of the major behavioral suggestions offered by the CIS, as recorded in the Call Record Form, and the behavioral actions actually taken by the callers, as recorded in the User Survey.

Behavioral Influences

In considering all possible influences on subsequent action, just over half (51.5%) of the general public callers felt that the CIS was "very important" in influencing their behavior. This substantial, but relatively lower percentage than for other groups, is not surprising given the results of the second question, which queried the general influence of additional information sources.

Of ten possible options, 46.5 percent of the respondents said that mass media (TV, radio, newspapers, magazines) influenced their behavioral actions. Relatives and friends were listed as the second most influential sources by 36.3 percent of the respondents. All other options influenced less than 15 percent of the respondents.

The general public was the only user group for whom indirect contact was more influential in behavior change than direct, personal contact. These data imply that mass media is a most influential means of reaching the general public, and that a variety of other sources are marginally influential.

Summary

As predicted from our model and the review of the previous literature, the general public appear to be passive information seekers. If a cancer message happens to catch their attention, and it is most likely that they see the message on television, it might stimulate them to engage in a limited information search, perhaps motivating them to call the CIS and request more information and, at least they report, actually read the information. That cancer message is more likely to be a catalyst for action for women, more educated, and white consumers than it is for men, less educated, and minority consumers. For most of those who actively enter the search process and choose the CIS as an information source, the information goal seems to be how to prevent cancer, particularly focusing on smoking.

In general, the cancers of greatest concern to the public seem to be breast, colon/rectum, and lung, although there are some differences in interest between the sexes and among the age, education, and ethnic groups examined. The saliency of these cancers probably results from their high incidence and attention by the media. As we predicted, this group's information searches seem to be abbreviated. Their calls to the CIS are shorter than calls for other groups and they are less likely to have called the CIS before. They report high levels of satisfaction with their CIS experience but the source they report to be most influential on their behavior is the mass media. The key to reaching this segment of the audience seems to be stimulating the initiation of the search process, since it is unlikely they will initiate the search themselves. Once they begin the process they seem likely to follow through at least to the step of reading printed literature sent to them. Given the pessimism and fatalism surrounding cancer, it is critical that these people be reached with accurate knowledge because the underlying beliefs about cancer formed at this stage of their involvement will affect preventive behaviors as well as their reaction if the disease becomes a personal threat.

6

Symptomatic People's Search for Cancer Information

This chapter focuses on those people (or their families/friends) who are experiencing some physical symptom which, at least in their minds, might be associated with cancer. The category does *not* include people who are at high risk but not symptomatic, nor does it include people who have a diagnosed non-cancerous condition, such as fibrocystic disease.

Based on the model of the information acquisition process presented in Chapter One, we would expect that this group's information search would be stimulated by the uncertainty that the symptoms themselves create. However, the way in which the person interprets the meaning of the symptom may be just as important. A message from the media or from another person might suggest that a previously ignored symptom could be a warning sign of cancer and create enough uncertainty to initiate the information search. For these people, the cost-benefit analysis might be the most critical step in our information acquisition model. For example, if the person's anxiety is low and the attitude toward cancer hopeful, the person might conclude that the benefits of further investigation warrant the cost and continue their search for information. However, most of the previous research on symptomatic people has focused on the well-documented delay between experience of a symptom and seeking medical care.

Delay in Seeking Treatment

People with symptoms that might mean cancer frequently do not seek medical attention immediately (Goldsen, Gerhardt, and Handy, 1963). For example, the average time of delay for women with breast cancer in Harlem was 10 months (Adams and Kerner, 1982). These delays can be quite critical since many types of cancer are much more likely to be cured if discovered and treated early. Thus, researchers have been quite interested in identifying factors which contribute to these delays.

A common assumption is that fear causes the delay. Green (1976) reviewed the literature on cancer delay and concluded that the relationship between fear and delay is not a simple one. For example, fear apparently interacts with knowledge about the significance of cancer symptoms in such a way as to increase delay when fear is intense, but to reduce delay when fear is low. Knowledge and belief in the efficacy of cancer treatment also decrease delay (Green, 1976). Eardley (1974) found that 74 percent of women studied reported that actions to seek care were affected by their knowledge of the benefits of early medical attention. Green (1976) also discovered that delay increased when symptoms were superficial lesions as opposed to internal lesions/masses, and decreased when symptoms were viewed as serious, unusual, or painful. Other researchers have examined demographic characteristics of symptomatic persons as predictors of delay. Antonovsky and Hartman (1974) found that those who delayed seeking medical treatment were of lower socio-economic status, had less education, and were older.

Another significant issue with symptomatic persons is what sources they consult during the period when they are trying to interpret their symptoms and decide what action they should take. Suchman found in 1965 that about three-fourths of a sample from New York state reported discussing their symptoms with some person other than a health professional before seeking formal medical care. This use of a lay referral network has been criticized for perhaps contributing to delays in seeking treatment.

Miller studied this issue in 1973 with 139 head and neck cancer patients. He found extensive use of a lay referral network. Sixty-two percent of these patients had consulted medically uninformed persons before seeing a physician, 26 percent had consulted medically informed persons (e.g., nurse or doctor who was a friend or neighbor) and only 12 percent had gone directly to a physician. Miller (1973), however, did not conclude that these lay consultations caused delays but instead believed that they were a positive force in convincing people to get medical attention. Miller did discover some differences in the use of lay referrals based on his deliniations of social class. Upper and middle class symptomatic people were more likely to consult only spouses before seeking professional treatment. The lower classes, if suspecting cancer, were less likely to discuss their symptoms with anyone else. One man explained:

> I didn't want to worry anyone. What my wife and friends didn't know wouldn't hurt them . . . anyway, I didn't want to bother anybody with my problems." (Miller, 1973, p. 957).

For perceived minor symptoms, the upper and middle classes used more medically informed sources; but for acute illnesses, the majority first turned to medically uninformed sources. Finally, the lower classes followed lay advice more frequently than did the upper or middle classes.

The CIS itself is an example of a medically informed source that symptomatic people can use to help them resolve uncertainties about their symptoms. Altman (1984) assessed the ability of the CIS to get undiagnosed, symptomatic callers to seek appropriate medical attention. (Only 2.3% of his sample were later diagnosed as actually having cancer.) He found that 75 percent of his sample contacted a health professional after their CIS call. One woman described her reaction to contacting the CIS, "She [the information specialist] left me feeling less afraid, which was something I didn't think would happen. I was too afraid to go to the doctor. After I spoke to her, I went." (Altman, 1984, p. 329). The callers' decision to follow the CIS advice to seek medical attention seemed to depend on the extent of their support network, their knowledge about cancer, and their financial coverage for health care costs. Of those people with health insurance 79 percent contacted a physician, compared to 62 percent of those without insurance.

In summary, symptomatic people are uncertain about their health status and many take considerable time to decide what action to take, time which may dramatically decrease their chance for cure in the case of cancer. Most of these people consult their own interpersonal networks as they attempt to make sense out of the symptoms they are experiencing. There is evidence that significant others often encourage them to get the medical attention they need.

CIS Calls from Symptomatic People

Who are the Callers?

Callers are classified as symptomatic when they call about symptoms that cause them concern about cancer but that have not been diagnosed by a physician. People in this category are further classified according to whether or not they have seen a physician. These symptomatic people placed 6.7 percent or almost 84,000 calls to the CIS during the four years covered in this analysis. About half of these symptomatic people had seen a physician before making the call and half had not. Another 1.5 percent of the calls to the CIS or about 19,000 calls were made by family and friends of symptomatic persons. In many cases, family and friends call the CIS because the symptomatic person is avoiding further information. For example, a young Hispanic woman called about her husband who was resisting seeing a physician because of fear of cancer and financial concerns, even though he was forgetting things, sleeping a lot, getting angry suddenly, and having headaches. A mother of another symptomatic person called the CIS because her daughter had a breast lump which a physician had told her to have biopsied three months earlier and the daughter had done nothing.

Although in general, three females with symptoms call for every male, there are striking gender differences between those symptomatic persons who have seen and have not see a physician before calling. The typical preponderance of female callers sharply increases for symptomatic people who have seen a physician, with 83.7 percent of all these calls made by females. Perhaps this disproportionately large number of female symptomatic callers who have seen a doctor can be explained by the large number of breast cancer calls. The initial visit to the doctor usually stimulates many questions about diagnostic procedures and treatment options. For example, a young female college student saw her doctor about a dark growth on one of her nipples. Her doctor referred her to a surgeon but she had to wait three weeks before she could get an appointment. She called the CIS to see if the time delay was critical and what other steps she could take while she was waiting. Perhaps males are more satisfied with their visit to a physician and less likely to continue an information search about their symptoms after seeing a physician.

By comparison, the symptomatic callers who have not seen a physician have gender patterns of CIS use similar to those for the general public, two female calls for every male call. More younger symptomatic people (under 30 years) who have not seen a physician call the CIS (32.2%) than those who have seen a doctor (17.8%). Perhaps the younger symptomatic people are less dependent on physicians for information and willing to try alternative sources. Otherwise, the age distribution of these callers is quite similar to the distribution for the general public. These callers, like the general public callers, tend to be better educated. About 50 percent of all symptomatic callers have at least some college education, compared to 30 percent of the total United States population.

Minorities are underrepresented in these symptomatic callers just as they are for the general public callers. An exception is blacks who have not seen a doctor, who represent 12.3 percent of the total symptomatic callers who have not seen a doctor. This proportion is more than the proportion of blacks in the general public callers (8%) and even more than the proportion of blacks in the total United States population (11.5%). There are two plausible explanations for this finding. One reason may be that blacks may not have personal physicians as often and rely more on emergency rooms or clinics for medical treatment. Therefore, when symptoms are discovered, they may first turn to sources of information other than a physician. An alternative explanation is that special CIS promotions have been targeted to blacks more heavily than to other minority groups, so they may be more stimulated to call.

What Do These Callers Ask About?

It is not surprising that the subject asked about most frequently is symptoms, but there is a dramatic difference for those who have seen and not seen a physician, as Figure 6.1 shows. Those who have not seen a physician are twice as likely to ask about symptoms as those who have seen a physician. Those who have seen a doctor are more likely to ask about diagnostic tests, general cancer information, and treatment. Apparently those who have not seen a physician are at a more preliminary stage of information seeking. They are most interested in the immediate symptoms they are experiencing. On the other hand, those who have seen a physician are, for the most part, beyond interest in the symptom and more concerned about next steps in the process such as diagnostic tests and treatment.

There were no gender differences for symptomatic people who had not seen a physician, but there were some male/female differences for symptomatic persons who had seen a physician. Males were more likely to ask about symptoms (44.5%) than were females (33.7%), but females were more likely to ask about diagnostic tests (29.8%) than were males (21.3%). Males may be seeking confirmation of their doctor's evaluation of symptoms while females may accept that evaluation more readily and shift their concern to the next stage in the process—diagnostic tests.

For both groups of symptomatic callers, as age increased more questions were asked about diagnostic tests, local organizations, services/physician referral, and treatment. These trends make sense since the older the symptomatic people, the more likely it is that they have cancer and need to be concerned about these issues. The reason for the one trend

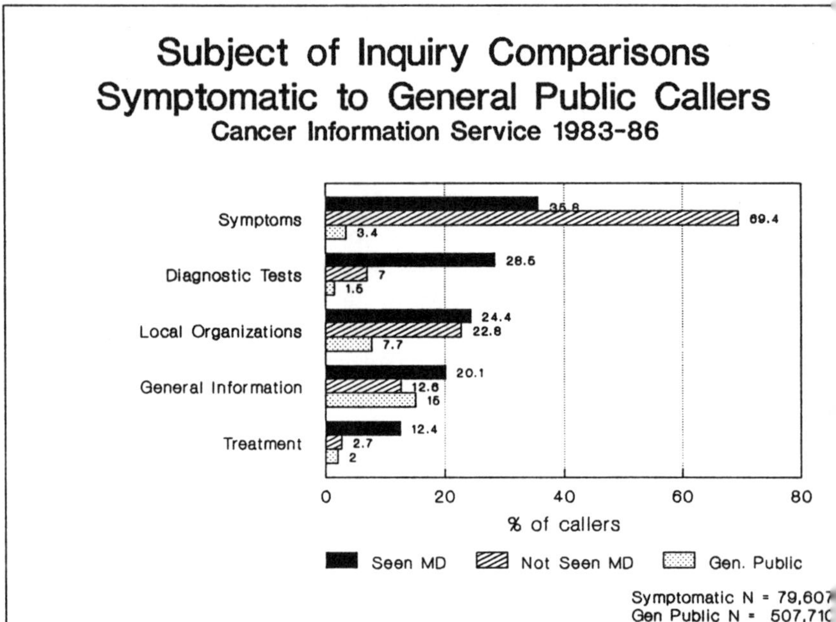

Figure 6.1

in the opposite direction is less apparent. The younger the caller, the more likely the questions focused on symptoms (72.4% of the callers under age 19 asked about symptoms while only 40.2% of those over age 60 asked about this subject). We might speculate that the younger callers have been exposed to more health information and are more conscious of the state of their own health, or that the constant attention in the media to cancer may have created a higher level of fear and concern about the disease among younger people than is warranted by their actual cancer risk. For example, a thirty-one year old male called the CIS anxious about possible lung cancer because of constricted breathing, even though he just recently had an x-ray that showed no tumors and had quit smoking. He seemed relieved when the information specialist pointed out the possible relationship between constricted breathing and other health factors, such as emotional upheaval. Another example is a male caller in his twenties who recently had many x-rays as a result of a car accident; he was feeling tired now and worried about the possibility of cancer since his mother had had breast cancer.

Questions about treatment increase with education but questions about symptoms decrease. Perhaps the less educated callers focus their questions on their most immediate needs—the actual symptoms they are experiencing—while the more educated callers project their concerns beyond the symptoms to other steps in the process. For example, a female in her thirties with only some high school education asked about the lump in her breast which her doctor had told her was just a cyst.

Hispanics in both groups asked more questions about local organizations and services and physician referral than other ethnic groups. This finding again reinforces the Hispanics' lack of access to medical care. Blacks in both groups questioned their immediate symptoms more often and asked about diagnostic tests less often than other ethnic groups. Symptomatic Asians asked more questions about general cancer information than other ethnic groups. Asians who had not seen a physician asked many more questions about diagnostic tests than other ethnic groups. This finding further reinforces the emerging picture of the Asian caller as one who is already very well-informed and asks sophisticated questions.

What Cancer Sites Were Asked About?

This discussion of sites must be prefaced by making it clear that the way this data set is constructed does not allow us directly to associate sites asked about with the site of the symptoms. In other words, a caller could have digestive symptoms and ask about colon/rectum cancer, but in the same call also inquire about lung or breast cancer. As for the general public, breast is the site most frequently asked about, followed by colon/rectum for both symptomatic groups. These two groups diverge, however, for the third most inquired about site. The symptomatic callers who have seen a physician rank cervix as the next subject but those who have not seen a physician have non-melanoma skin cancer in third place. Since cervical cancer usually produces no symptoms in its early stages, callers asking about cervical cancer are likely to have been told by their physician that their pap test was abnormal. On the other hand, skin changes are symptoms easily recognized by individuals.

Another interesting difference between those who have and who have not seen a physician is the frequency of questions about colon/rectum. Although it is the second most inquired about topic for both groups, almost twice as many questions are asked about this site by those who have not seen a doctor (21.2%) than by those who have seen one (11.2%). Perhaps, because there are so many reasons for gastro-intestinal problems, there are many people experiencing symptoms who are uncertain about the causes. Those who have already seen a physician may have been reassured that their symptoms were not likely to be cancer. For example, a man in his sixties who had not seen a physician called the CIS about stomach problems he had experienced for some time. He wanted to know if his symptoms were serious and what were the symptoms of stomach cancer.

As we would expect, more than half of all questions from symptomatic women were about breast cancer. It is interesting, though, that, unlike the other sites, more questions about breast cancer were asked by those symptomatic women who had seen a physician than by those who had not seen a physician. The frequency of questions by this group may reflect the uncertainty women face about treatment options for breast cancer. Almost three times as many questions about colon/rectum cancer come from males as from females. Finally more questions about lung cancer come from male symptomatic callers than their female counterparts.

Age seems to have a relatively limited impact on site of inquiry. The only consistent trend is for colon/rectum questions to increase with age, from only 8.9 percent of the questions from those under 19 to 20.5 percent of the questions from those 60 and over.

For several sites, (i.e., breast, melanoma of the skin, non-Hodgkin's lymphoma, and Hodgkin's disease) the number of questions increases for the better educated symptomatic caller. This trend is consistent with the pattern repeated frequently in the literature that the more educated segments of society are the most aggressive information seekers.

Another pattern in these data, however, contradict that viewpoint. More questions about lung and colon/rectum cancer are asked by the least educated callers. Lung cancer questions can probably be explained by the higher incidence of smoking in the less educated segments of the population. It may be that the less educated callers are less knowledgeable about gastro-intestinal problems and therefore have greater uncertainty when they experience these symptoms and so ask more questions about them.

Ethnicity affects the relative frequency of site questions for symptomatic callers in ways similar to the general public callers. Black symptomatic callers ask more questions about cervical cancer than most other ethnic groups and those who have seen a physician ask three times as many questions about this topic as those who have not seen a physician. Like blacks, Hispanic symptomatic callers who have seen a physician ask four times as many questions about cervical cancer than those Hispanic symptomatic callers who have not seen a physician. Perhaps many of these calls are stimulated by women receiving abnormal pap smear results.

Hispanic symptomatic callers ask fewer questions about lung cancer than other ethnic groups. Those who have not seen a physician ask more questions about breast cancer, a pattern also seen for Hispanic general public callers, which may reflect a greater anxiety about breast cancer in this ethnic group.

Symptomatic Asians do not have any specific patterns for site inquiries; the number of American Indians is too small for trends to emerge.

How Did the Callers Learn of the CIS?

Although television is the most frequently cited source of information about the CIS for both groups of symptomatic people (20.6%), the telephone book is a very close second with 19.4 percent. These results indicate that while many symptomatic people learned of the CIS from a more passive source, an equal number used a more active source. The data cannot tell us, however, whether those symptomatic people who reported television as their source learned about the CIS before experiencing a symptom and retrieved that information when they initiated their information search or whether they had ignored the symptoms until some message on television prompted them to take action.

There were no gender patterns for source of information about the CIS for either group of symptomatic people. For both groups the reliance on television decreased with education. The use of newsletters/magazines and brochures/pamphlets/books increased with education only for those who had not seen a physician. These results corroborate generally recognized media usage patterns; that is, the more educated the user, the greater use of print media and the less use of electronic media, especially television.

Analyzing sources of information by age demonstrates that for all symptomatic people, the use of newspapers increases consistently as age increases, from a low of 3 percent for callers under age 19 to 8.2 percent for those 60 and over. The only other significant finding appeared in the use of television for those under age 19. They are much greater users of television than other age groups.

For all symptomatic people, each minority group reported television as their source of information about the CIS more often (an average of

28.7%) than the group of whites (20.8%). Blacks and Hispanics reported the highest use of television and Hispanics reported the highest use of radio. Asians were most likely to report the use of brochures/pamphlets/ books.

Description of Responses to Calls

Behavioral Suggestions

About two-thirds of all symptomatic people (66.5%) were advised to talk to or visit a physician. The second most frequently offered behavioral suggestion was to read literature sent; 31.1 percent of symptomatic persons who had seen a physician were given this advice compared to 21.3 percent of the symptomatic persons who had not seen a physician. This difference seems logical in that people who have not yet seen a physician are less certain about their condition, and hence it would be more presumptuous to send them a booklet on a specific type of cancer. For symptomatic persons who had seen a physician, 24.1 percent were encouraged to seek a second opinion, whereas only 4 percent of callers who had not seen a physician were given this advice. Again, these discrepancies between groups seem appropriate; one would expect generally that only those people who had already seen a physician would be more likely to be told to get a second opinion. Callers who had not yet seen a physician might also get this advice as a general recommendation.

The only other difference between the two groups was in the proportions referred to NCI-sponsored cancer centers. For those who had seen a physician 11.8 percent were referred, compared to 5.2 percent for those who had not seen a physician. These percentages are low, probably because none of these callers had confirmed diagnoses of cancer. This difference also seems appropriate, in that referrals to specialists usually occur after consultation with a primary physician.

For symptomatic callers who had not seen a physician and who did not have a personal physician, more males (22.0%) than females (14.6%) were advised to talk to or visit a physician.

For both groups of symptomatic people there is a pattern of more sophisticated referrals being given to the most educated groups. Figure 6.2 illustrates this pattern. Referrals to NCI or specialized cancer centers give callers access to the state of the art in treatment, including clinical trials. There are two explanations for these results. First, the more educated callers ask more sophisticated questions and may directly prompt

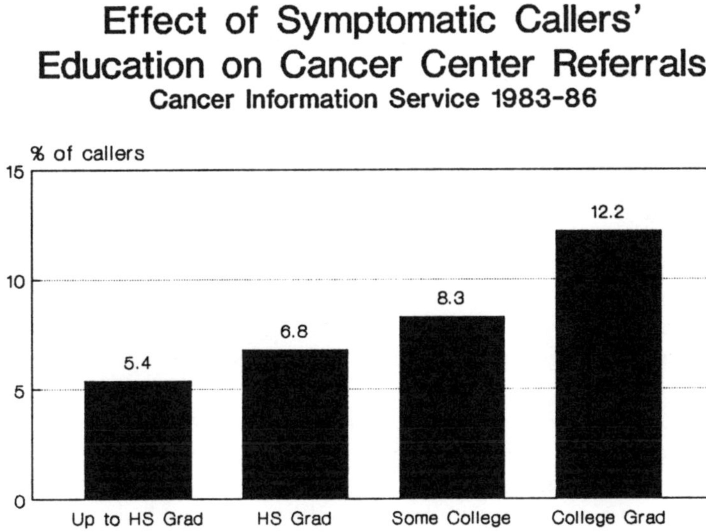

Figure 6.2

these referrals by asking about experimental treatments. The second explanation is that the CIS information specialists, consciously or unconsciously, adapt their responses to their perception of the caller's educational level. In either case, these results demonstrate a potential problem with the system that warrants additional scrutiny. Everyone who calls, regardless of educational level, should have equal access to the best information and treatment available.

Time on the Phone

More time is spent on the phone with symptomatic callers who have seen a physician than with symptomatic callers who have not seen a physician. For example, 63.0 percent of calls from those who had not seen a physician were short (1–5 minutes) compared to only 40.1 percent of those who had. Perhaps those callers who have not seen a physician are quickly handled by a referral to a physician. These time patterns seem to be contrary to what would be desirable. When symptomatic people call who have not seen a physician, it is an ideal time to prepare them for the visit to the doctor with appropriate questions to ask. People with symptoms may also be experiencing a powerful cue-to-action (an event which serves as a catalyst for change), and hence it would be a productive time to recommend related lifestyle changes such as stopping smoking.

Follow-Up to the Phone Inquiry

Symptomatic callers who had seen a physician were more likely to receive some type of follow-up (44.5%) than were symptomatic callers who had not seen a physician (37.8%). For both groups, the follow-up almost always consisted of sending publications. Most follow-up was handled in five minutes or less. The time required for follow-up was consistently greater for symptomatic callers who had seen a physician than for those who had not.

For both groups of symptomatic callers, women are more likely to receive some follow-up than are men. Moreover, that follow-up usually takes more time for women than for men. Hispanics are the ethnic group most likely to receive follow-up in the form of publications.

User Response to the CIS

User Satisfaction

This group of callers recorded the highest overall rate of satisfaction with CIS services at 95.9 percent, with 83.9 percent being "very satisfied." Another 2.8 percent were "neither satisfied nor dissatisfied," 0.8 percent expressed that they were "somewhat dissatisfied," and 0.5 percent were "very dissatisfied."

A high rate of having one's "most important question answered by the CIS" may account for the high rate of satisfaction. Slightly more than 87 percent, more than general public or patient users, affirmed that their most important question was answered.

Behavioral Response

It is interesting to note that on average, symptomatic persons and their families and friends were slightly more active in behavioral change than either of the other two groups of callers. The uncertainty of cancer for them may be a catalyst for increased action.

Table 6.1
Comparison of Behavioral Suggestions with Actions Taken
Symptomatic Callers (user survey respondents)

Behavioral suggestions/actions	Percent told	Percent did
Read materials sent	69.7	78.9
See personal physician	53.8	24.9
Referred clinic/physician/hospital	17.9	6.8
Seek second opinion	11.8	16.8
Share information with others	9.9	58.0
Referred agency/service	3.4	5.7
Learn self-detection techniques	2.9	16.7
Stop/reduce smoking	2.5	12.0
Reduce exposure to environmental health hazards	1.3	5.3
Change eating habits	—[a]	4.1

[a]Although 4.1 percent reported a change in eating habits, this category is not specifically listed under behavioral suggestions on the CRF.

In only two areas were actions taken to a much lesser degree than recommended by CIS. Over half of these callers were recommended to see their personal physician, and nearly one fourth reported doing so. About 18 percent of the callers were referred to a clinic, physician, or hospital; only 6.8 percent actually contacted these sources. One reason for this lack of action was summed up by a respondent:

> I think the CIS is great because of its convenience, and also it is not as costly as a trip to the family physician. The information I obtained . . . answered my questions precisely.

Table 6.1 compares CIS suggestions with users' behavioral actions.

Behavioral Influences

This group of callers listed the CIS as having the highest rate of importance in influencing behavioral change (63.8%). The influence of additional sources was consistent with those for cancer patients and their family/friends. Forty-two percent listed relatives and friends as influential; 30.6 percent cited their physician; 19.3 percent recorded the mass media, and less than 14.0 percent was attributed to other sources.

Symptomatic persons and their family/friends were a group whose behavior was influenced by a wide variety of sources, particularly interpersonal ones.

Summary

Given the great uncertainty faced by someone who is experiencing a symptom he/she suspects may be cancer, it is surprising that this type of caller is responsible for such a small percentage of calls to the CIS. Perhaps this low level of usage of the CIS by symptomatic persons is further evidence of the delay phenomenon among cancer patients. It is particularly frustrating that those who are most likely to delay in seeking medical treatment for a symptom—the poor, the uneducated, and the elderly—are also the most infrequent users of the CIS. Moreoever, that frustration is exacerbated by realizing how much potential the CIS has for combating this delay phenomenon. When symptomatic people do call the CIS and are referred to physicians, Altman (1984) reports around three-fourths of them actually follow through on this advice. Our data show that figure to be lower, at 46 percent. Altman's study included more extensive follow-up of his sample of callers, including telephone interviews, which may account for his higher figure. The CIS also offers many advantages over other information sources these people tend to turn to. The CIS is free, unlike a visit to a clinic or a physician; the CIS offers authoritative and anonymous information, unlike advice from friends and families.

Those symptomatic people who do call are demographically quite similar to the general public caller in that they are more often female, white, and educated. Blacks, however, who are symptomatic and have not seen a doctor use the CIS proportionately more frequently than any other group of black callers.

Symptomatic callers ask about the subjects most salient to them, for those who have not seen a doctor, symptoms; and for those who have seen a doctor, diagnostic tests, general cancer information and treatment. These callers, like the general public callers, ask most often about breast and colon/rectum cancer followed by cervix and non-melanoma skin cancer. These data suggest that the most uncertainty about cancer symptoms may surround colon/rectum symptoms.

Although television is still the source most frequently reported by symptomatic callers, it is closely followed by the telephone book. This finding suggests that symptomatic people may be divided into two groups: those who are not aware of the CIS but who respond to their symptoms by becoming aggressive information seekers and look in the telephone book for information sources; and those who ignore or repress their symptoms until stimulated by a compelling message on television.

These callers are most frequently told to visit or talk to their physicians. In fact, the CIS cannot diagnose the symptoms over the telephone, so this advice seems appropriate. Moreover, the information specialists at the CIS can often help locate inexpensive and appropriate medical care if the caller needs it.

Apparently the symptomatic caller is quite satisfied with his/her CIS experience. This group of callers reports the highest rate of satisfaction, the most behavioral change, and the highest rating of influence for the CIS of any group of callers examined.

For those symptomatic people who call the CIS, the symptom itself, a changed perception of it, or the urging of friends or family is probably the stimulus that initiates the information search. However, the small number of these callers suggests that many symptomatic people may be deciding that the "costs" of the information may exceed the benefits. Therefore, the key to reaching these people may be messages emphasizing the importance of early attention to symptoms coupled with an optimistic outlook for survival.

7

Cancer Patients' Search for Cancer Information

This chapter focuses on cancer patients and their families and friends, for whom a diagnosis of cancer is a powerful stimulus, creating an intense need for information. We would predict that the cancer patient and family/friends would recycle through the information acquisition process repeatedly as new uncertainties arise, stimulating the search for new information. The motivation for continual searches probably depends on the perceived benefits from earlier efforts. If the patient believes the information helped him/her make informed choices and gain control, then another search is more likely. If, however, the patient experienced frustration by inability to get information or to interpret contradictory information, then the costs may appear too great to try another search. Unfortunately, the previous literature suggests that many patients are dissatisfied with their information seeking attempts, particularly those involving physicians.

Desire for Information

Patients usually report dissatisfaction with the amount of information they are able to get about their illness. Ley (1980) reviewed several surveys of patients' satisfaction with communication with their physicians. Based on the U.S. studies reviewed, the median percent of patients who were dissatisfied was 36 and the range of dissatisfaction was from 8 to 51 percent (Ley, 1982, p. 341). Waitzkin (1985) confirmed this patient dissatisfaction, saying that patients tend to be more dissatisfied about the information received from their physicians than any other aspect of medical care except high costs and waiting time. A Hodgkin's disease patient expressed this dissatisfaction vividly when he said:

> A curious patient can always find scraps of information; I noticed that my blood-test card had "HD stage IVB" scribbled on it—how much more distressing to seek the meaning of this in an outdated medical dictionary than to have it set in proper context by a knowledgeable and sympathetic doctor. (p. 613).

Ley (1982) reports considerable evidence of patients' desire for as much information as possible about their illness. Ironically, however, patients' expressed desire for information does not always determine their behavior. Numerous studies have shown that patients do not actively seek information from their physicians. Boreham and Gibson (1978), for example, interviewed 80 female patients prior to consultation and discovered that they did *not* have a high level of knowledge concerning either their diagnosis or treatment yet expressed a strong interest in gaining such information during the consultation. Even though the consultation immediately followed this interview highlighting their information needs, these women still did not question the physicians directly. In fact, whatever information they were told was determined almost totally by the doctors. Only 27 requests for information were made in these 80 consultations.

This general desire for information from physicians also applies to cancer patients. A study assessing both surgeons' and breast cancer patients' viewpoints on information seeking (Messerli, Garamendi, and Romano, 1980) found that 86.2 percent of breast cancer patients had unanswered questions at the time of the mastectomy. For those women who did not ask all of their questions, "not knowing what to ask" and "being too emotionally upset at the time" were the primary reasons for their reticence. Cassileth, Zupkis, Sutton-Smith, and March (1980) interviewed 256 cancer patients to determine their preferences for information and participation in their care preferences. Despite strong age differences, a majority of patients in each age group wanted detailed information and preferred active participation in their own care. Moreover, information enhanced rather than destroyed their hopefulness. Similarly, Rainey (1985) found in a study of the effects of preparatory education for radiation oncology patients that a large majority of patients read the booklet provided and that 85 percent responded affirmatively to the item, "I would like to learn more about radiation therapy."

Some authors have attempted to account for differences in information seeking behaviors with demographic characteristics. Social class frequently has been suggested as a predictor of how much information patients desired. Waitzkin (1985), in his review of information giving in medical care, concluded that lower class patients want as much information as higher class patients but may not have as much success in getting it. Boreham and Gibson (1978) did find a relationship between some demographic characteristics and desire for information. People who sought detailed information versus those who avoided it were younger, white, and better educated. Younger patients defended their information seeking with such comments as: "It's my body and my disease," "You have to take responsibility for your own body," and "Ignorance is fear." Not knowing about one's disease was often associated with uncertainty and unrealistic fears, a condition patients described as "worse than not knowing the facts." A typical justification for their preference for minimal information from older patients was: "I'm not qualified," or "I need as little to worry about as possible." (p. 833).

There are suggestions in the literature, however, that cancer patients' desire for information may be influenced by two other factors—the personal coping style of the patient and the stage of disease the patient is experiencing. Schain (1980) suggests that patients do better when the intensity of information they receive is consistent with their coping strategy. Two types of patients are identified by Schain—"monitors and blunters." Schain describes a monitor in the following way:

> if a woman comes into the office for a breast biopsy with a pad, pencil, small tape recorder, and carrying Rose Kushner's book, *Why Me*, one can feel fairly confident that this woman is what is termed a "monitor" or information seeker. (p. 1038).

Blunters, on the other hand, are usually meek or stoic, appear uninformed and do not seem to want to know very much. Although Schain does not speculate on the proportion of patients who may be monitors or blunters, a study by Cassileth, et al. (1980), in which people receiving radiation therapy were asked if they wanted more information about the therapy, may suggest these proportions. Most (about two-thirds) of the patients did want more information; even those who knew a lot felt uncertain and wanted confirmation of their information. But one-third of these patients responded that they did not want more information. Orr (1986) found that 18 percent of the 51 breast cancer patients who were interviewed repeatedly during the first year after mastectomy tried to avoid any cancer-related information. More patients showed partial denial or some reality distortion. For example, 35 percent said that they would prefer not to know a negative prognosis. These studies suggest that up to a third of cancer patients may be blunters.

The stage of disease that the cancer patient is experiencing also may explain his/her desire for information. Abrams (1966) identified three stages which cancer patients might experience: (1) the initial stage, when cancer has been verified by clinical evidence; (2) the advancing stage, when metastases or the spread of cancer is confirmed; and (3) the terminal stage, when the condition is considered irreversible. In the initial stage the mood is optimistic and there is direct and truthful communication. If the cancer patient enters the advancing stage, the mood becomes tense and anxious and the patient seldom confronts the physician for information. The communication between patient and physician becomes measured, considered, and guarded as the patient becomes more and more dependent on the physician. If the disease progresses to the terminal stage, little communication of any kind occurs, especially in the areas of greatest anxiety. Perhaps in this terminal stage, the patient does not ask or is too ill to ask, or the physician has too much anxiety and avoids communication. Information is not as important as the presence of another person to help ease the feeling of abandonment. Stage of disease as a predictor of information acquisition also was supported by Gotay (1984). She interviewed female patients in early and late stage cancer and their mates and found that seeking more information was ranked second as a coping strategy for early stage patients (third for their mates) and eleventh for late stage cancer patients (twelfth for their mates).

Patients' Understanding and Recall of Information

Even if physicians do inform their patients, patients may not be able to understand or recall the information after the consultation. Based on her own studies and a review of the literature in this area, Bertakis (1977) estimated that outpatients forget as much as one-third of what the doctor tells them. Ley (1972b) argued that the amount of information forgotten depends upon the amount presented, thus patients presented with five, ten, or fifteen statements would be expected to forget approximately two, five, and seven statements. Pendleton (1983) rejected these earlier estimates of forgetting, accusing them of poor methodology and oversimplification. He used data from 84 appointments in a general practice and found different levels of recall depending upon the type of information being presented. Instructions regarding medications produced an 83.8 percent recall, "things to do" advice resulted in a 76.3 percent recall, and 61.5 percent of general information items were recalled. In this study, the quantity of information negatively affected recall of only the latter two categories. Although Pendleton found that physicians gave less information to low socio-economic status patients, the lower social classes tended to recall the information as well as middle classes.

Evidence of this recall problem comes from three kinds of research: (1) patients' own reports of not understanding, (2) indirect assessment through the readability of patient educational materials; and (3) direct tests of patients' comprehension of information given by physicians (Ley, 1982).

Patients' Reports

Patients frequently report that they have not understood what their doctor has told them. Table 7.1 summarizes some of the studies done by Ley and his associates (Ley, 1982) which show the percentage of patients reporting that they do not understand what their general practitioner has told them.

Readability of Patient Educational Materials

An indirect assessment of patients' understanding is possible by measuring the reading level necessary to comprehend a particular printed patient educational material. Several standard readability formulae exist, for example the Flesch Reading Ease formula, the Dale-Chall formula (Ley, 1982) and the SMOG and Fog indexes (Freimuth, 1979). These readability measures yield a score which indicates, in terms of grade level, the reading ability required to understand the material. Table 7.2 shows an example of applying the SMOG index to several patient education materials as well as articles in lay magazines (Freimuth, 1979). Since 60 million people, almost one-third of adult Americans, read at

Table 7.1
Patients' Reported Failures to Understand What Their General Practitioner Had Told Them

	Percentage not understanding			
Investigation	Diagnosis	Etiology	Treatment	Prognosis
Kincey, et al. (1975)	7	17	14	13
Ley, et al. (1975)	47	47	43	53
Ley, et al. (1976b)	30	43	—	35

Source: From P. Ley, Giving information to patients in J. R. Eiser (ed.) (1982). *Social Psychology and Behavioral Science* (Chichester: John Wiley & Sons, Ltd.), p. 344. Reprinted with permission from John Wiley & Sons, Ltd.

Table 7.2
SMOG Grade of Lay Publications and Patient Pamphlets

Publication	SMOG grade
Ebony	
"A Simple Test for Breast Cancer"	11
Reader's Digest	
"What Smoking Does to Women"	12
Ladies Home Journal	
"Cancer Therapy Everybody's Discussing"	14
Newsweek	
"Kids with Cancer"	10
Washington Post	
"What You Should Know About Cancer"	15
National Cancer Institute's Site-Subject Pamphlets	
Malignant melanoma	11
Breast cancer	11
Skin cancer	13
Leukemia	14
Fox Chase Cancer Center	
Facts about breast cancer	12
Mammography: What you need to know	14

Source: From V. S. Freimuth (1979). Assessing the readability of health education messages. *Public Health Reports*, 94(6), 568–570.

less than a ninth grade level (Kozol, 1985), most of these materials are going to be too difficult for much of the public to comprehend.

Direct Tests of Patient Comprehension

The most valid evidence of the problem patients have in understanding and retaining information comes from those studies that directly test patient comprehension. For example, Ley (1972a), in trying to explain why some information was recalled and some forgotten, discovered that both primacy and saliency of the information were positively related to recall. In other words, patients remembered best that information which was given early in the consultation and/or was most important to them. Other researchers attempted to manipulate some aspect of the information in order to increase recall. Ley, Bradshaw, Eaves, and Walker (1973) found that explicit organization of the information increased patient recall. Patient restatement of key points conveyed in the consultation followed by physician feedback increased retention from 60.8% to 83.5%

of the key points (Bertakis, 1977). Written information was another strategy that successfully increased information gain (Ellis, Hopkin, Leitch and Crofton, 1979).

Recently, however, researchers (Tuckett, Boulton, and Olson, 1985) have taken a more sophisticated approach to this issue and instead of just measuring quantity of information recalled, have examined three levels of response to information: recall, interpretation, and commitment. They discovered that most difficulties with the information arise not from failure of memory, but at the stages of interpretation and evaluation. Specifically, they discovered that one in ten patients could not recall key points on at least one topic, but that one in four patients could not make correct biomedical sense of the key points, and nearly one in four patients were not committed to the key points made by the physician.

Patients' sense of what their doctor told them depended on their own construction of biomedical ideas. Commitment to the physician's advice seemed to depend on the extent of education of the patient, the nature of the diagnosis, and the patient's own explanatory model. The less educated the patients, the less likely they were to share the doctor's assumptions. The more unusual and threatening the diagnosis, the more likely the patients were to stay with their own theories about the illness. Finally, the more discrepant their own explanatory model was from the physician's and the stronger their attachment to it, the less positively they evaluated the doctor's views. In addition, mothers often demonstrated strong belief in their own theories about their child's illness and were reluctant to agree with a physician's theory if it was different from their own. Similarly, minority ethnic group members often persisted in their folk interpretations of medical problems rather than accept the physician's biomedical explanation. These problems in accepting information again reinforce our concept of the public as active participants in information processing, constructing new information rather than passively receiving it.

Effects of Information

Waitzkin and Stoeckle (1972) identified five positive effects resulting from physicians' communicating information about patients' illnesses; (1) enhances the accuracy of history-taking; (2) provides more useful medical records; (3) increases patients' compliance with therapeutic regimens; (4) increases patients' satisfaction; and (5) improves patients' physical and psychological responses to therapy.

History-Taking

The patient's ability to provide an accurate account of past illnesses and treatments depends on the quality of information he/she received at the time. If a physician explains an illness completely and accurately to a patient, that complete communication feeds back to the physician the next time he/she has to take a history on that patient.

Medical Records

Medical records should indicate what information was transmitted to patients during their visits. If records do not contain this information, patients are often given contradictory information which leaves them confused, angry, or dissatisfied. This problem is especially acute in hospital settings where many care-givers attend to each patient.

Patient Satisfaction

Patient satisfaction is at least partially dependent on the information the physician chooses to communicate. Mitchell and Glicksman (1977) found that over one-half of their sample of patients in radiotherapy "remembered receiving *no* helpful information about their treatment" from the referring physician. In pediatric practice, dissatisfaction of parents was greatest when they failed to get the information about causation and the nature of the illness that they expected to get from the doctor. (Korsch, Gozzi, and Francis, 1968).

Patient Compliance

An estimated one-third to one-half of all patients fail to follow fully the treatment prescribed for them (Stone, 1979). Cancer patients are no exception. Evans and Clarke (1983) reviewed the records of patients who entered a hematologic-malignancy unit at a Los Angeles County hospital during 1978 and 1979 and found that only 25 percent could be considered active cases. A total of 20 percent refused treatment; another 15 percent of patients moved (which may be covert refusal since many were Hispanics who believed that cancer was untreatable and wanted to go home to die); the remaining 40 percent had died.

Stone (1979) reviewed the compliance literature and concluded that there is a consistent positive association between amount of instruction given by the physician and adherence to the physician's expectations. Moreover, there is a positive correlation between information and satisfaction and between satisfaction and compliance. Therefore it is likely that increased information will indirectly increase compliance to a point. Ley (1983) constructed a simple model to show the relationships among understanding, memory, satisfaction, and compliance. Ley explained the relationships in the following way:

> Whether patients will comply with advice will depend in part on whether they have understood and remembered what they have been told, and on their level of satisfaction with communications. In turn satisfaction with communications will be partly dependent on memory and understanding. Finally understanding should affect the probability of information being recalled. (p. 95).

This model predicts that:

1. Increases in understanding will lead to increases in satisfaction and compliance.
2. Increases in memory will lead to increases in satisfaction and compliance.
3. Increases in satisfaction will lead to increases in compliance.

For example, there is considerable evidence to support these predictions. Hulka, Cassel, Kupper, and Burdette (1976) found that patients who recalled information that their physicians had told them about their illnesses had lower error rates in following recommendations. Not all the research in this area supports the positive relationship between information and compliance. The investigation by Sackett, Haynes, Gibson, Hackett, Taylor, Roberts, and Johnson (1975) found that compliance was unaffected by learning about hypertension and its treatment, even when the information was completely mastered. Ley (1979) reported two experiments which also showed that information does not necessarily affect weight loss. Although there is evidence to support the positive relationships among understanding, recall, satisfaction, and compliance, there appear to be other unexplained factors sometimes distorting these positive relationships.

Therapeutic Outcomes

Researchers also have examined the effects of giving patients information on such therapeutic outcomes as reduction of pain, reduction of anxiety, and length of hospital stay. Ley (1977) reviewed most of these studies of the effectiveness of preoperative communication in reducing postoperative distress. Table 7.3 summarizes the effects of three kinds of information: (1) technical instruction, e.g., how to breathe, how to cough; (2) informational, e.g., what procedures would be used, and when; and (3) quasi-psychotherapeutic, e.g., letting the patient express anxiety and fears. In 10 of 11 studies, preoperative communication was able to shorten hospital stay an average of two days. In 7 of 9 studies, patients exposed to preoperative communication required fewer painkillers (analgesics).

Apparently these positive benefits of communication accrue even indirectly through patients' family members. Skipper and Leonard (1968), for example, studied the effects of detailed information procedures in dealing with parents of children who undergo tonsillectomy. Their research confirmed that children with better informed parents have more rapid recovery as reflected in a number of physiologic measures.

Not all the research in this area supports the hypothesis that more preparatory information results in improved therapeutic outcomes. Miller and Managan (1983) divided 40 gynecological patients about to undergo a colposcopy, a diagnostic procedure, into "monitors" and "blunters" and gave them voluminous preparatory information. Subjective, physiological, and behavioral measures were taken before, during, and after the

Table 7.3
Effects of Preoperative Communication on Postoperative Progress (Number of Studies)

Type of communication	Analgesic requirement: Fewer	Analgesic requirement: Same	Days in hospital: Fewer	Days in hospital: Same
Instruction	1	1	2	0
Information	3	1	3	1
Quasi-psychotherapeutic	1	0	2	0
Mixtures of the above	2	0	3	0
Summary	7	2	10	1

Source: P. Ley, Giving information to patients in J. R. Eiser (ed.) (1982). *Social Psychology and Behavioral Science* (Chichester: John Wiley & Sons, Ltd.), p. 344. Reprinted with permission from John Wiley & Sons, Ltd.

procedure. While high information did not result in less anxiety and arousal, it apparently did result in slightly fewer overt behavioral signs of pain. The ability of information to reduce the behavioral signs of pain is supported by several other studies (e.g., Egbert, Battit, Welch, and Bartlett, 1964; Johnson, 1973; Johnson and Leventhal, 1974; Staub and Kellett, 1972; Johnson, Fuller, Endress and Rice, 1978; and Johnson and Rice, 1974).

While previous research consistently shows some desirable outcomes from preparatory information given to patients, these outcomes differ depending upon the nature of the information, and the type of effects measured. The most consistent relationship seems to be the positive effect of sensory information on behavioral signs of pain.

Information Acquisition by Families of Patients

Although much has been written about the process patients use to acquire information, the information acquisition process for patients' families has largely been ignored. Yet a diagnosis of cancer creates uncertainty for the family member just as it does for the patient. There is evidence that family members have even greater difficulty acquiring information than do patients.

In interviews with members of cancer patients' families, Krant and Johnston (1978) asked whether family members talked to the doctor. Only 9 percent of the family members reported that they talked freely with the physicians; 46 percent said that they did not talk at all to the physicians. In fact, 40 percent of those interviewed could not even identify the physician presently in charge of the case. Only 59 percent of the family members were given the diagnosis of cancer by the physician and 15 percent remained angry about the way in which they were told. In a study (Barbarin and Chesler, 1984) of seven empirically distinct dimensions of staff behavior relevant to their relationships with parents of children with cancer, information transmission independently predicted more of the individual satisfaction measures than any other single behavior.

Another study (Wright and Dyck, 1984) in which family members of hospitalized cancer patients were interviewed found that difficulty getting information was mentioned first as a concern by 16 percent of family members. Another 49 percent mentioned this problem when probed for additional concerns. Specifically, these family members spoke of difficulty getting concrete answers from doctors, getting in touch with doctors, getting information from doctors by telephone, or finding out about the patients' daily progress from nurses. Family members perceived that the amount and nature of information was controlled by the health care team, particularly the physician. Moreover, family members reported that lack of access to this information increased the uncertainty and anxiety experienced by them and the patient. Family members' highest score on a needs scale was to be kept informed of the patient's condition. These needs were reported to be the highest when the patient had experienced a recurrence of the cancer. Wright and Dyck (1984) described the crisis nature of recurrence as follows:

> At this stage, families realize that the much-hoped-for cure has not occurred, and doctors and patients reach a communication impasse thus isolating patients (and families) from the health team and increasing their anxiety. (p. 373).

Northouse (1986) suggested three reasons for the limited contact between health professionals and family members of cancer patients. First, family members are seldom in the hospital when physicians make their rounds. Physicians usually make rounds in the morning and family members generally visit in the evening. Second, family members are expected to initiate any contact which occurs with physicians, and many family members are hesitant to bother a busy physician. Third, both family members and physicians appear to minimize the importance of the physician-family relationship. Both family members and physicians seem to believe that the patient is the primary focus and that family members' needs are somehow less legitimate. As a result, few formal channels of communication are established to meet the family members' needs for information, forcing them to rely on second-hand information from the patient.

Summary

The most extensive body of literature on searching for health information can be found for patients. Patients generally are dissatisfied with the amount of information they receive from their physicians. Even though most patients typically want as much information as possible, they are reluctant to ask their doctors for this information. Cancer patients' desire for information may be influenced by their own coping style and by the stage of disease they are experiencing.

Even if patients are able to get information from their physicians, they may not understand it or recall it. There are many positive effects of information which is understood and remembered. Information can enhance the accuracy of future history-taking and the quality of medical records. It can heighten patient satisfaction and compliance. Moreover, information can reduce pain, anxiety, and length of hospital stay.

Patients' families appear to have more difficulty getting information than do patients. Several reasons for this lack of communication between doctors and patients were suggested.

CIS Calls from Cancer Patients and Their Family/Friends

Given the difficulties family/friends report in finding accurate, appropriate, and timely sources to meet their health information needs, it is not surprising that they have placed about 22 percent of the calls to the CIS over the last four years. It is surprising, however, that only 11 percent of the calls to the CIS in the last four years have come from cancer patients themselves. What we may be seeing are family/friends acting as information agents for cancer patients. Unfortunately, the data we have available do not allow us to determine whether the family/friend callers are seeking information for their own edification or to pass on to cancer patients. An examination of some verbatim reports on the call record form, however, suggests that both objectives often motivate a call. For example, a woman, whose father has asbestos-related lung cancer that has metastasized, was going to visit him and was quite anxious about what to say to him. In addition to her own needs, she also asked for advice for him on hospitals and dietary treatments. In the following sections of this chapter, we will present a basic description of these cancer patient and family/friend callers and the nature of their questions.

Who are the Callers?

The 33.5 percent of the CIS callers who are patients and family/friends of patients are very similar demographically to the general public callers described in Chapter Five. As might be expected, however, they are more likely to have called the CIS before; 30.6 percent of patient callers and 25.3 percent of family/friend callers have called the CIS before contrasted to only 8.8 percent of the general public callers.

Three female patients and their family/friends call for every male even though the incidence of cancer in males and females is not this disproportionate (two females for every male). The patients and family/friends who call the CIS are more educated than the general public callers

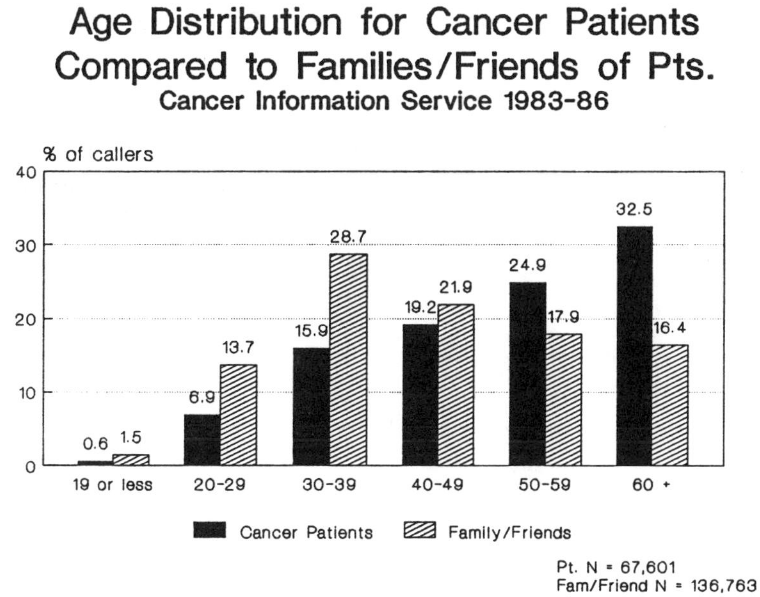

Figure 7.1

and the U.S. population. More of the family/friend callers have at least some college (60.4%) than patient callers (54%).

Figure 7.1 shows the age distribution of patient callers compared to family/friends. Patient callers are consistently older than family/friend callers. Twice as many patients as family/friends are 60 or over. This trend is a mirror image of the cancer population, that is, cancer patients tend to be older people. Twice as many family/friends are 30–39 years old, suggesting that younger family/friend callers may be adult children calling for their parents. It is clear that in some cases the decisions on treatment are made by an entire family. For example, a woman from California in her forties called the CIS about her mother-in-law who had bronchial cancer and had been advised to have "radiation to her head" by an oncologist. The caller reported that the whole family was divided on whether this treatment should be done and if it was necessary. The caller's brother had just died from cancer and she felt rather fatalistic about the disease. Her father was scared of making a choice.

Minority cancer patients and family/friends of cancer patients are even more underrepresented than they are in the general public calls to

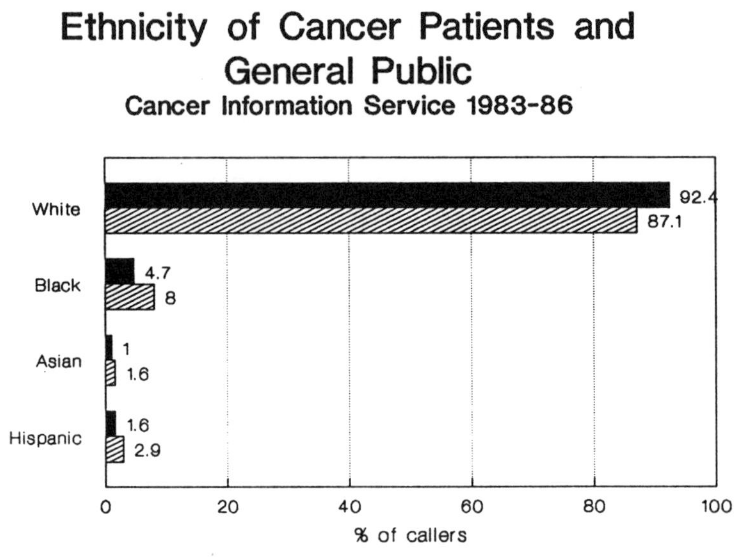

Figure 7.2

the CIS. Figure 7.2 shows the percentages of cancer patients compared to general public callers.

The underrepresented ethnic groups are even more striking considering that blacks, for example, have a higher rate of incidence and mortality for cancer than whites (American Cancer Society, 1987). Hispanics have a lower incidence and mortality rate than other ethnic groups which may be due to the relative youthfulness of this group (one-third of Hispanics are under the age of 15) or to the incomplete status of Hispanic data collection (American Cancer Society, 1987).

What Do These Callers Ask About?

The subjects patients and family/friends ask about differ greatly from questions for other groups of callers. They have a diagnosed cancer, so risk factors, prevention, and screening are less important to them. What is important are treatment issues, local organizations and services including physician referral, and general cancer information. (See Figure 7.3.)

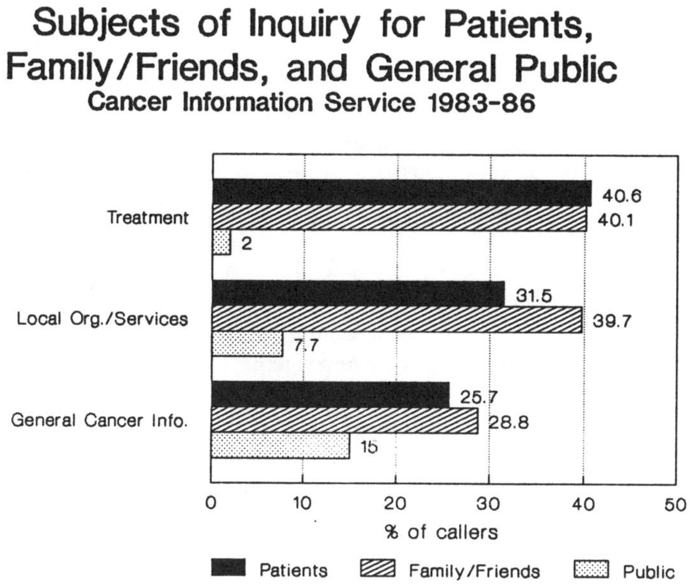

Figure 7.3

Many of the treatment questions imply dissatisfaction with a physician's recommendations. For example, a female caller from Oklahoma who had a bladder tumor and had had chemotherapy was not satisfied with her doctor's recommendation that her bladder be removed. She called the CIS to learn where to go for treatment. Some of the treatment inquiries seem to be prompted by another information search in which the caller became aware of a new treatment. For example, a woman in her fifties called about her husband who was undergoing chemotherapy. She wanted to know about laser surgery. Another male caller in his fifties had read about interferon and called to ask if it might be used to help his wife who had cancer.

Many of these treatment questions reflect the lack of communication between patients and physicians. For example, a female friend of a cancer patient called because the physician had said that it was not possible to determine based on scans whether tumors on her friend's spine had shrunk. The caller was asking if this were true and if so, why? A female caller in her fifties complained that the doctors "don't answer questions." A male caller in his fifties who had had surgery and radiation a year earlier for a brain tumor but was now having trouble walking said, "the doctor doesn't tell me anything. He says everything is fine but it's not."

When these subjects of inquiry are analyzed for the different demographic characteristics of cancer patients and their family/friends, only a few differences emerge. More men ask about treatment issues than do women for both cancer patients and family/friends of cancer patients. Treatment questions increase as education and age increase. Moreover, whites and Asians ask about treatment proportionately more often than do the other ethnic groups.

These results suggest that older, well-educated, white and Asian males are more aggressive information seekers about their own or a friend or family member's cancer treatment. The traditional explanation that women function as information agents for their families receives only partial support from these data. Instead, these results suggest that a more complex model may be necessary to explain these gender patterns. There is ample evidence from the health care literature that women are less aggressive patients than are men. Perhaps they are also less aggressive information seekers when it comes to searching for information that may challenge the medical establishment, i.e., treatment issues.

What Cancer Sites Were Asked About?

Table 7.4 shows the five cancer sites most frequently asked about by these cancer patients and family/friends of cancer patients. Almost half of the patient inquiries (46.2%) were about breast cancer while one-fifth of family and friends asked about this site. On the other hand, 21.1 percent of family/friends' inquiries were about lung cancer but only 8.5 percent of patients inquired about this site. In general, when family/friends call proportionately more often than patients about a site, it appears to be because cancer in that site is more serious or survival is lower

Table 7.4
The Five Cancer Sites Most Frequently Asked About for Cancer Patient Callers and Family/Friend Callers

	Cancer patients	Family/friends
Breast	1	2
Colon/rectum	2	3
Lung	3	1
Prostate	4	5
Melanoma of skin	5	7
Leukemia	8	4

(e.g., lung, brain, and pancreas cancer), or it is a cancer that frequently affects children or young adults, e.g., leukemia and Hodgkin's disease. In either case, family and friends seem to be acting as the patient's information seeker. Often there is real desperation in these calls. For example, a woman from Florida whose husband's cancer had been called inoperable called to ask, "What do we do?" Another caller, a patient herself, was told by her physician that her cancer had metastasized to her lungs and that nothing could be done, and was calling to ask if that were true.

Three times as many inquiries about sites came from women as from men for both patients and family/friends. This disproportionately high number of inquiries from females is more striking when one realizes that the incidence of cancer for women is roughly twice that for men. Clearly women cancer patients inquire more about specific sites than do men. Gender influenced inquiries about sites in an expected way for cancer patients, e.g., almost all of the breast, uterus, and cervix questions were from women while almost all of the prostate questions were from men. These patterns of gender differences did not emerge in analyses of inquiries about sites from family/friends. Instead, all these results followed the familiar pattern of three times as many inquiries from women as men.

We did find a relationship between the amount of education and the sites most frequently inquired about. For lung, cervix, and uterine cancer, the proportion of inquiries from cancer patients decreased as education increased (see Figure 7.4) but for melanoma of the skin that trend was reversed for cancer patients, with inquiries increasing as education increases. The negative relationships are particularly striking because they reverse the persistent trend of more calls coming from the most educated segments of the population. These relationships are expected, however, because there is a higher incidence of both lung and cervical cancer among individuals of lower socio-economic status. It is not clear why the positive relationship for melanoma exists. An analysis of the inquiries by age of the caller yields only the obvious anticipated relationship. Types of cancer sites which affect younger persons are inquired about more by this age group. For example, 19–29 year olds call more often about leukemia and Hodgkin's disease.

Table 7.5 shows the rank order for sites inquired about by each ethnic group. The breast was the site most frequently asked about for all the ethnic groups, with nearly half of the questions in all groups except American Indians, where it was about one-third. Around 10 percent of all site questions concerned the colon/rectum; this was the second most frequent site of inquiry for whites and Asians but third for blacks, Hispanics, and American Indians. The cervix was in second place for blacks

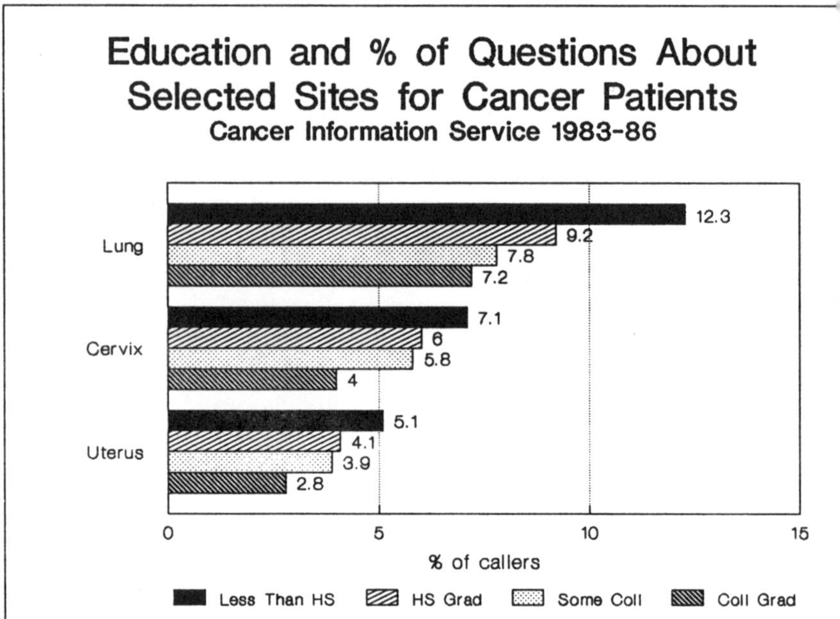

Figure 7.4

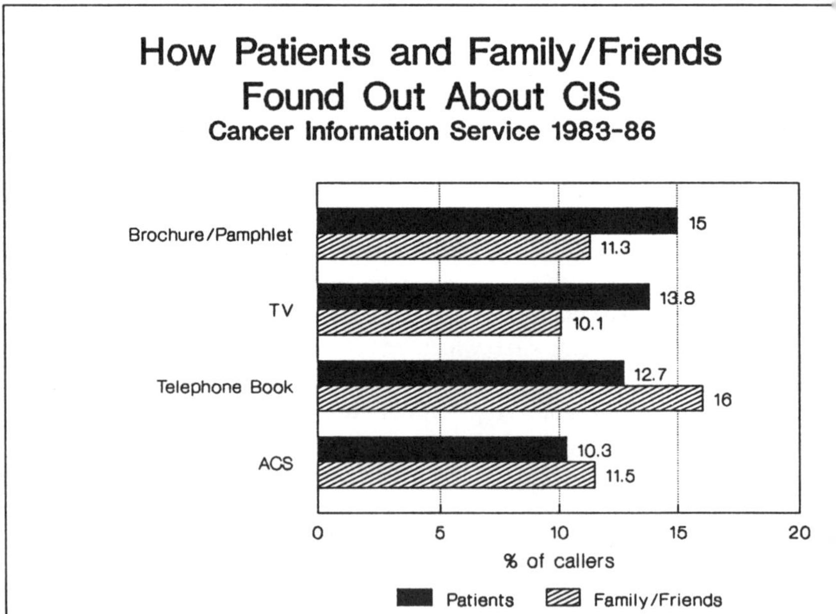

Figure 7.5

Table 7.5
Rank Order of Sites Inquired About by Different Ethnic Group Callers
Cancer Patients

	White	Black	Asian	Hispanic	Amer. Indian
Breast	1	1	1	1	1
Colon/rectum	2	3	2	3	3
Lung	3	4	4	5	4
Cervix	7	2	6	2	5
Uterus	9	5	3	4	2

and Hispanics but much lower for whites and Asians. The uterus was high on the American Indian and Asian list but lower for blacks and whites.

How Did the Callers Learn of the CIS?

There is more variability in how patients and family/friends first learn about the CIS, with these two groups showing less dependence on television than other CIS users. Figure 7.5 shows the sources mentioned by these two groups of CIS callers. Both these groups, but especially family/friends, seemed to search more aggressively for cancer information than did the general public. These active searchers relied more on intermediaries such as the telephone book, the American Cancer Society, and brochures and pamphlets, than on television. Educational level was the demographic characteristic which seemed to most influence source of information about the CIS. For both patients and family/friends of patients, the less educated callers were more likely to learn about the CIS through television. (See Figure 7.6.) The age group that seems unique in its source of information about the CIS is the youngest group of callers, the teenagers. Over 32 percent of teenage patient callers and 37.7 percent of family/friend callers in this age group report television as their source. By comparison an average of only 14 percent of patients and 12 percent of family/friend callers from the other age groups report television as their primary source.

As is the case in several studies which examine ethnicity and health information sources, Hispanic patient callers report television as their source of information about the CIS more frequently (25.1%) than do the other ethnic groups (who range from 12–19 percent). The same trend appears for Hispanic family/friends of cancer patients, but the differences are smaller.

Education of Callers Who Found Out About CIS from TV

Cancer Information Service 1983-86

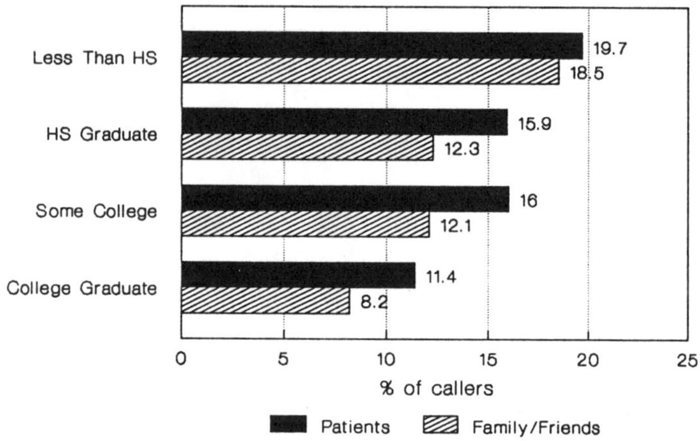

Figure 7.6

Education of Callers Referred to Specialized Cancer Center

Cancer Information Service 1983-86

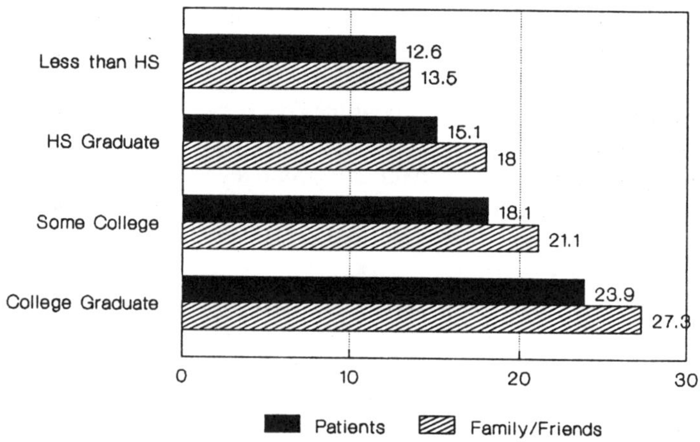

Figure 7.7

Description of Responses to Calls

Behavioral Suggestions

About 32 percent of patients and family/friend callers were advised to talk or visit with physicians and to read literature. 12.7 percent of the patient callers and 8.5 percent of the family/friend callers were advised to seek a second opinion. About 23 percent of patients and family/friends were referred to NCI or a specialized cancer center. As might be expected, about five times as many family/friends were told to share cancer information obtained with other persons than were patients.

Teenage patient callers were given different advice from other age groups. It was less frequently suggested that they seek a second opinion or go to NCI or a specialized cancer center. In addition, teenage family/friend callers were less likely to be counseled to go to a cancer center. Callers in this age group were more likely to be asked to read literature.

Male callers and more highly educated callers (both patients and family/friends) were more likely to be referred to a specialized cancer center. (See Figure 7.7.)

These results highlight a continuing dilemma for information systems. The "information rich" are more likely to be aware of the service, to know how to use it, and to actually use it. Consequently the gap widens between the information "haves" and "have nots." Moreover, this inequity is exacerbated by the system's response. Like the rest of society, the information specialists who answer the CIS phones are likely to adapt their information to their perception of the gender and educational level of the caller. Most often this adaptation is probably appropriate and indeed exemplifies the important "personal" component of this information system. It is possible, however, that some personal biases of the staff may interfere with the quality of the information disseminated.

Time on the Phone

In general, calls with patients and family/friends took more time than most other calls. Around 14 percent of these calls took more than 15 minutes, compared to only 1.5 percent of the calls from the general public. About 40 percent of the calls with these two groups of users took 1–5 minutes and slightly over 40 percent took 6–15 minutes. There appeared to be a relationship between education and time on the phone to handle the inquiry for family/friends but not for patients. Less time was spent with less educated family/friends. It is possible that these callers asked less complex questions. Thirty-seven percent of calls from college graduates, but 47 percent of calls from those without high school diplomas, took only 1–5 minutes.

Calls from teenagers tended to be shorter than calls from other age groups for both patients and family/friends. Almost 58 percent of calls from teenage cancer patients were only 1–5 minutes compared to an average of 37 percent from cancer patients of other ages. The same pattern existed for family/friends of cancer patients.

Follow-Up to the Phone Inquiry

Sending publications was the most frequent follow-up for the half of these groups who required any follow-up. About half of all cancer patients and family/friends of cancer patients were sent publications. About 4 percent of both cancer patients and family/friends of cancer patients were called back.

Most of the calls which required follow-up could be handled in 1–5 minutes. Only 8 percent required more than 6 minutes.

User Response to the CIS

User Satisfaction

Just over 80 percent of patients, their family, and friends were "very satisfied" with the CIS. Altogether, over 95 percent expressed satisfaction with the CIS, 2.7 percent were "neither satisfied nor dissatisfied" and less than 2 percent were dissatisfied. The high rate of user satisfaction among patients, their family and friends may frequently be a result of explanations which provide callers with an understanding of their condition:

> I have now had surgical conization, and I was more at ease because I was able to except (sic.) and understand what was going to be done to me.

A more dramatic illustration of user satisfaction came from the Woods family in Kentucky (McLain, 1985). Leah Woods, a ten-year-old girl, had been diagnosed with osteosarcoma, a cancer of the bone. All the cancer experts in their area recommended the same procedure, amputation of the leg. But Mike and Kathy Woods, Leah's parents, were not satisfied with that option. Mike located the CIS number in a book of toll-free numbers he had picked up on sale from his local book store. Linda Linville, an information specialist at the Kentucky CIS, took the Woods' call and told them of a limb salvage program. In this experimental procedure, the diseased bone is removed and replaced by a titanium steel rod similar to a car jack. As the child grows, the rod is extended. "Linda sent us everything she had on it," Woods said. "We got the names of the doctors, their hospitals, a nutrition booklet, lists of American Cancer Society services, and even where the Ronald McDonald Houses were located." (McLain, 1985, p. 8.)

The family arranged a visit with Dr. Michael M. Lewis at the Hospital for Joint Diseases in New York and Leah was accepted as only the sixth child to receive the experimental implant. The operation was successful and the family returned home. Leah still faced a year-long series of chemotherapy treatments during which she lost her hair and suffered prolonged bouts of nausea. Now two years later, Leah walks straight and tall on both legs. The Woods family remember the night they found the telephone number. Kathy described her call to the CIS, "It was the answer to a prayer." (McLain, 1985, p. 9).

Behavioral Response

A significant 83.5 percent of these callers reported reading the material(s) sent to them. Only 10.3 percent contacted their physicians, whereas 32.0 percent were advised to do so. An even smaller percentage, 7.3 percent, contacted a referred agency or support group service, compared to 18.7 percent who were advised to. However, a larger group than recommended, 16.8 percent compared to 10.2 percent, sought a second opinion. One respondent commented on the value of such an action:

> My husband has Castleman's Disease. I spoke to the doctor at Johns Hopkins. He was very nice and put my mind at ease. I also received a letter from Johns Hopkins explaining the disease and the reasons I should see an oncologist. This too was very reassuring.

All other behavioral changes involving self-motivation rather than any outside contact exceeded the proportion of CIS suggestions. Table 7.6 provides the percentage breakdown of suggestions and corresponding actions taken.

Table 7.6
Comparison of Behavioral Suggestions with Actions Taken
Cancer Patients (user survey respondents)

Behavioral suggestions/actions	Percent told	Percent did
Read materials sent	64.5	83.5
See personal physician	32.0	10.3
Referred clinic/physician/hospital	24.9	6.4
Referred agency/service	18.7	7.3
Share information with others	15.9	61.9
Seek second opinion	10.2	16.8
Learn self-detection techniques	.8	6.5
Reduce exposure to environmental health hazards	.8	5.0
Stop/reduce smoking	.4	5.6
Change eating habits	—[a]	12.5

[a] Although 12.5 percent reported a change in eating habits, this category is not specifically listed under behavioral suggestions on the CRF.

Behavioral Influences

Over 60 percent of patients, their families, and friends, responded that the CIS was "very important" in influencing health behavior actions.

Of the ten possible sources of influence on their health behavior, 49.6 percent cited relatives and friends as influential; 23.5 percent cited their physician; and only 13.5 percent recorded the mass media as influential. Interpersonal contacts were clearly more influential in behavior change for cancer patients and family/friends than for the general public.

Summary

As predicted from our model and the previous literature, cancer patients and family/friends are the most aggressive information seekers of any of the groups we have examined. They rely on more active information sources such as the telephone book, the ACS, and other people more than on the passive mass media. Moreover, they are more likely to be repeat users of the CIS. As Dervin predicted in her theory of information, these callers do have gaps in their understanding of what is happening to them or ones close to them and ask questions to close those gaps. Consider the caller who doesn't understand why her mother-in-law, after having a bone scan, was being sent to an orthopedist instead of an oncologist.

Most of these information gaps concern treatment issues, local organizations and services, and general cancer information, as evidenced by the subjects of inquiry for these callers. The cancers of greatest interest to these callers are breast, lung, and colon/rectum—the same cancers as the other groups reported.

There also is evidence from these calls that the information-seeking process is sometimes a collective one with whole families getting involved, each finding pieces of information and together deciding on interpretations. Family and friends have their own information needs too. Often these needs concern communication issues—what to say to terminally ill loved ones, how to tell someone he or she has cancer, and how to get information and respect from care givers.

Demographically, patient and family/friend callers are very similar to the other two groups of callers, i.e., more frequently female, white, and well-educated. Patient callers tend to cluster in the older age ranges (50 plus) while family/friend callers are frequently younger (20–40 years old).

The CIS most frequently advises these callers to read literature sent and/or see their physicians. While almost one-fourth of these callers are referred to NCI or a specialized cancer center, there is a potential equity problem in those referrals. The data reveal a tendency for males and well-educated callers to be referred to these centers more often. These calls also take more time than calls from any other group of users.

These CIS users were highly satisfied with the service but did not report as much satisfaction as did symptomatic callers. Patients and family/friends followed or exceeded the CIS advice for reading literature and seeking a second opinion, but did not comply as frequently with such advice as seeing their physician, going to a clinic or hospital, or contacting a local agency or service.

Patients and family/friends rated the amount of influence the CIS had on their health behavior higher than did the general public, but lower than did symptomatic callers. Interpersonal sources were clearly more important to these callers than to the other groups examined.

An examination of the specific content and language used in a sample of these questions from the call record forms reinforces the conclusions from the literature review in the first part of this chapter. Most of these callers are dissatisfied with the information they are receiving from their physicians, and many also express uncertainty about how to ask questions of their doctor. Perhaps some of these callers have been given answers by the doctors but have misunderstood or forgotten the information. The CIS gives them a chance to ask again, or to get material in writing that they can refer to over and over again. Those information seekers who do find and use the CIS report high satisfaction with their experience. This satisfaction is reinforced by the large numbers of these callers using the CIS more than once. Perhaps the reason for this satisfaction is that the CIS is one of very few information sources which allows the users to define their own information needs and responds to them in a highly personal and unique manner.

8

Stimulating Information Seeking

Promotion is an integral part of a comprehensive communication system such as the CIS. Those people who are seeking information about cancer must be aware of the CIS as a potential source of information before they can use it. Moreover, we know that some uncertainty must be experienced before individuals initiate a health information search. For some people, this uncertainty is created by their own physical symptoms. For others, however, the uncertainty must be stimulated by external sources, e.g., a television message, a poster, or a comment from a friend.

There is only limited data on what proportion of the U.S. population is aware of or has used the CIS. According to a Cancer Prevention Awareness Survey conducted by NCI between February and April 1985, 20 percent of the 1,898 people in the general population were aware of the CIS telephone number, (1-800-4-CANCER) while 30 percent of the 263 blacks sampled reported this awareness (National Cancer Institute, 1986). Only 2.8 percent of the general sample and 1.5 percent of the black sample reported ever using the service.

In this chapter, we will describe how both planned promotion and unplanned events can promote a comprehensive communication system like the CIS. Planned promotions are used to create awareness of the service and to stimulate information seeking on specific topics and from specific groups of people. For example, as a result of NCI's emphasis on smoking cessation, a series of PSAs on smoking cessation encouraged viewers to call the CIS for help in quitting. Other planned promotions frequently target specific audiences because they are underusers of the CIS (e.g., blacks) or because they have a higher risk of cancer (e.g., people over 50 years old). Unplanned events, such as news of President Reagan's colon cancer, must be responded to appropriately to maintain the credibility of the system and can become an opportunity to promote the availability of the system.

Planned Promotion

Use of Social Marketing

Social marketing techniques (Sciandra and Stein, 1983) can be the foundation of a comprehensive promotion plan. The basic premise of social marketing is to apply marketing concepts and techniques to the promotion of a socially beneficial cause rather than commercial products or services. There must be a balance between the product or service being offered and the needs and wants of the consumer. Cancer information, for example, is an offering that is not inherently desirable to many people. Different population segments vary according to their need for and readiness to accept the information and therefore require different strategies. The following marketing principles should be considered in the development of the plan:

1. Audience segmentation with a separate but complementary promotion strategy for each target audience.
2. Selection, when possible, of target audiences in a readiness stage most likely to respond to promotion.
3. Selection of channels appropriate to the target groups, including mass media, health professionals, and other intermediaries.
4. Use of positive, anxiety-reducing appeals delivered by sources credible to the target audiences.
5. Clarity through use of a single message, especially in broadcast advertising.

The early promotion activities of the CIS often proceeded without enough advance planning and with little research into effective messages and media to reach particular audiences. This lack of planning occasionally resulted in target groups chosen for CIS promotion that were those least likely to call the CIS. For example, in 1982, a public service announcement (PSA) was developed based on two key points: (1) the tremendous progress in the treatment of childhood cancer over the last ten years; and (2) calling the CIS for facts about cancer.

A beautifully produced 30-second television PSA featuring a mother and son was distributed nationwide, tagged with the CIS telephone number (see Figure 8.1). Pretesting results were impressive and bounceback postcards from public service directors indicated a very favorable response and strong intent to provide air time. The number of CIS calls in response to the PSA was a great disappointment—only a handful nation-

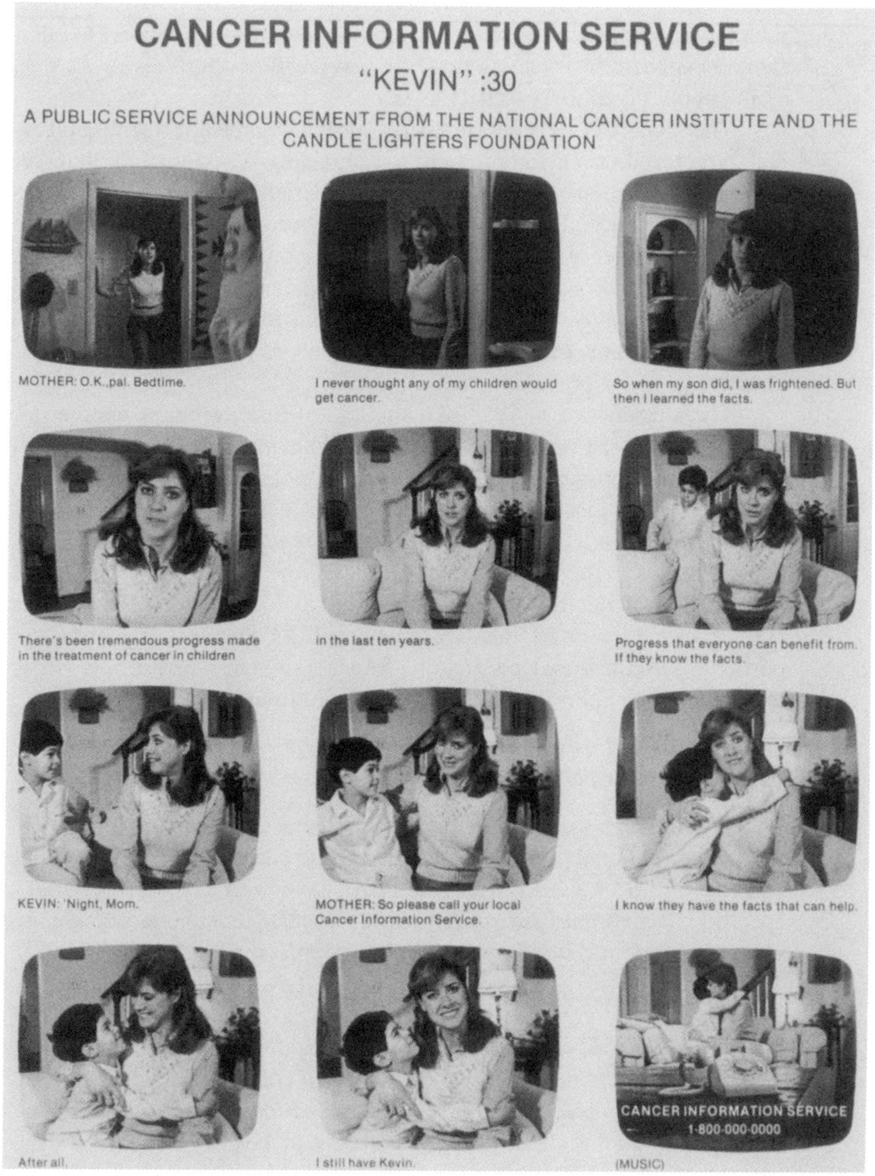
CANCER INFORMATION SERVICE
"KEVIN" :30
A PUBLIC SERVICE ANNOUNCEMENT FROM THE NATIONAL CANCER INSTITUTE AND THE CANDLE LIGHTERS FOUNDATION
MOTHER: O.K.,pal. Bedtime.
I never thought any of my children would get cancer.
So when my son did, I was frightened. But then I learned the facts.
There's been tremendous progress made in the treatment of cancer in children
in the last ten years.
Progress that everyone can benefit from. If they know the facts.
KEVIN: 'Night, Mom.
MOTHER: So please call your local Cancer Information Service.
I know they have the facts that can help.
After all,
I still have Kevin.
CANCER INFORMATION SERVICE
1-800-000-0000
(MUSIC)

Figure 8.1

wide. The lack of response may have been due to the relatively small number of people with a particular interest in childhood cancer. In addition, no specific instructions for action were offered to the viewer, they were simply urged to "call for the facts."

The marketing plan subsequently adopted by the CIS identified several target audiences for promotion campaigns based on literature reviews, focus group analyses, and past experiences. The initial groups identified for special promotion campaigns were smokers who want to quit, persons over 50 years of age, blacks, and cancer patients and their families. At least one CIS promotional campaign has now been targeted to each of the above groups. The design and resulting impact of some of these campaigns on the CIS will be discussed more fully later in this chapter.

The introduction in 1983 of a single, toll-free telephone number for the CIS, 1-800-4-CANCER, significantly enhanced the development of these national promotions. This and other technological enhancements to the CIS were discussed in Chapter Two. Customized call routing automatically forwards each call to the appropriate regional or national office, depending upon the area code of the originating call. The introduction of this telephone number eliminated the need for multiple tagging of public service announcements (PSAs) and presented new opportunities for national promotion. The mnemonic number was easily remembered by callers even for some time following exposure.

Television PSAs

Even though the CIS has used other channels to promote its service, most of the national promotion resources have been devoted to television, specifically PSAs. Generally, these PSAs have been developed around a specific cancer topic and message with the CIS telephone number included as an action step for obtaining more information.

The mass media, especially television, have always been seductive tools for health communicators because they offer the potential of reaching millions of individuals with important health information quickly and inexpensively. Yet the results of these health communication campaigns have often been disappointing. It is not uncommon for less than ten percent of the target audience to report seeing or hearing any of the campaign messages. A number of processes work to consistently narrow the audience for PSAs. Hammond, Freimuth, and Morrison (1987) presented a funnel model of the gatekeeping process which showed how a PSA with a potential of reaching over 170 million Americans may only be broadcast to 14 percent of homes with television sets, and be responded to by less than one percent of the potential 170 million. Even though a PSA may be distributed to all TV stations in the country, only a small percentage of these stations actually air the spot. The funnel narrows even further when the PSA reaches the audience, who selectively expose themselves to messages, avoiding exposure to messages that they have no interest in, or if exposure cannot be avoided, ignoring or selecting out only that portion of the message which reinforces their prejudgments, interest, and likes, or simply forgetting everything about the subject to which they have been forcibly exposed.

Exposure is only the first hurdle that PSAs must overcome. Flay, Ditecco, and Schlegel (1980) have described the causal chain which occurs between exposure to messages and behavior change:

> Exposure will lead to awareness, but only when the message is attended to.
> Awareness will lead to changes in knowledge, but only when the message is comprehended.
> Changes in knowledge will lead to changes in beliefs, but only if the arguments or conclusions of the message are accepted or yielded to.
> Changes in beliefs might lead to changes in attitude, intentions, and ultimately behavior.

Even if one accepts this explanation of the theoretical causal chain, controversy remains regarding where along this chain to measure for effects. One might argue that the further along this chain one measures the more important the effects. On the other hand, the potential effects of messages decrease as one measures further along the chain, as does ability to control extraneous variables. For example, PSAs promoting the CIS could be assessed at the level of increased awareness of the service itself. Or they could be measured using a criterion of increased knowledge about the CIS or the specific cancer topic being discussed. Or they could be evaluated based on the number of people who actually call the CIS in response to the PSA. Or the most stringent criterion could be used, i.e., did advocated health behavior change (e.g., smoking cessation) actually occur?

In spite of these measurement problems, there is evidence that PSAs can have positive effects. The Stanford Heart Disease Program was the first health education effort to demonstrate that the use of mass media alone (mostly PSAs) did have positive effects on the health behavior of a specified community (Maccoby and Solomon, 1981). A cautious optimism was expressed by Atkin (1979) in his review of mass mediated health communication campaigns. He concluded that "the use of mass media campaigns can produce modest influence on the health orientation of the audience." (Atkin, 1979, p. 664). A mass media campaign designed to increase public understanding of the dangers of asbestos exposure also showed positive results in awareness and attitude change among targeted groups (Freimuth and Van Nevel, 1981). Flay (1986) reviewed 39 program/campaigns designed to influence cigarette smoking and concluded that mass media programming can significantly effect smoking behavior.

Most health information campaigns do not rely on PSAs alone. The hypodermic needle model of mass media effects which depicted the media as capable of strongly and directly persuading the public, has been replaced with the multistep flow model, which suggests that information communicated by the mass media is filtered through many interpersonal contacts (Rogers, 1983). The promotion of the CIS fits this multistep flow model well in that the mediated messages about cancer which include the 1-800-4-CANCER number use mass media to stimulate the viewer to call the CIS which in turn provides the interpersonal component of the model.

Other Media

Although the primary focus of planned national promotion has always been television, other types of promotion have been used, with varying degrees of success, over the life of the CIS. One of the most effective ways of generating CIS calls has been a simple listing in the white pages of the telephone directory. As mentioned in a previous chapter, telephone directory listings accounted for 9.2 percent of CIS calls. Since the CIS is a federally-funded program, paying for inserts in the yellow pages of telephone directories has not been permitted, but might have generated additional calls. The important point to note about white page listings is that they must be placed in all directories in each area covered by a regional office. Since the telephone system in this country has been decentralized into many small telephone companies, it is necessary to contact each company individually and arrange for local directory listings.

Radio has been used to a limited extent in national promotions, accounting for 4.2 percent of CIS calls, but it has not been nearly as effective as television promotion. However, for targeted promotions, it may be a viable option. It is possible to target radio promotions quite effectively because the audience characteristics of radio stations are much more defined than for television. For example, a promotion targeted to blacks included, in addition to television PSAs, a series of radio PSAs that were sent only to radio stations that targeted their programming to black audiences. Although the numbers of calls generated through radio promotion was much smaller than for television, it may have reached individuals who would not have otherwise contacted the CIS and/or reinforced messages appearing in other media.

Posters also have been developed to publicize the CIS telephone number. Accounting for only 0.1 percent of calls, they are not a primary means of generating inquiries. Like radio, however, they have been viewed by people who did not learn of the CIS through other media and/or reinforced other channels. Posters can be placed in locations where a particular target audience is likely to view them, such as doctors' offices, churches, buses, or subways.

Print ads have been developed at the national level and been designed so that regional offices can add a local identification and distribute them to appropriate publications in their areas. These ads account for a portion of the 4.6 percent of calls generated through newsletters, newspapers, and magazines.

Promotion campaigns should consist of a variety of materials for a variety of media. A comprehensive promotion campaign might consist of several television PSAs of varying lengths, several radio PSAs, a series of print ads, a poster, and other materials. Distribution for some of these materials is best handled nationally, and others may be more effectively distributed through local channels.

In addition to promotion campaigns and materials developed nationally, regional offices may develop and produce materials for local promotion. In most cases, nationally developed materials are appropriate for local use, however, some regional programs may wish to target promotions to audiences that will not be reached by national promotions. For example, the CIS office in Hawaii has produced materials designed specifically for native Hawaiians.

The effective promotion of a comprehensive communications program is a complex, challenging task. The most effective promotions are carefully planned with characteristics of the target audience in mind.

Descriptions of CIS Planned Promotions

Each of the three CIS promotion campaigns described in the following sections provides an opportunity to study a unique aspect of promotion. The first campaign, a series of smoking-cessation PSAs delivered by the

U.S. Surgeon General, allows assessment of the impact of using a highly credible spokesperson. The second campaign, which included two television PSAs featuring Aretha Franklin, was targeted to blacks and presents a chance to assess the effectiveness of that targeting. The third campaign, a collaboration between Kellogg and NCI to promote fiber in the diet, offers us an unusual opportunity to see the effects of paid advertising on calls to the CIS.

The "Surgeon General" Public Service Announcement Campaign

Campaign development

The "Surgeon General" campaign, a collaborative effort between the NCI and the Office on Smoking and Health (OSH), resulted in a large, measurable public impact. For this campaign, it was decided to use a spokesperson to deliver the anti-smoking messages, each targeted to a specific audience: the confirmed smoker who has tried previously to quit but has now gone back to smoking; the family and friends of smokers; and the parents of children who are either smoking now or are potential smokers. Dr. C. Everett Koop, U.S. Surgeon General, was chosen as a spokesperson because his title appears in the warning box of every cigarette package produced in the U.S., he is the government's chief spokesperson when data are released each year on smoking and its effects on the public and, most importantly, he is perceived as highly credible and deeply committed to smoking cessation.

Description of the campaign materials

The integrated marketing communications program consisted of television and radio public service announcements, collateral print materials, and the CIS telephone number as a follow-up for obtaining information on local resources, answers to questions, and publications. The creative technique consisted of an interview or "news" format. The four PSAs resulted from Dr. Koop spending an entire day being interviewed by a skilled producer/director, sitting off-camera. This day's worth of questioning resulted in 4,000 feet of generic tape from which four 30-second announcements were developed.

The messages were very straightforward. For example:

> Dr. Koop: "After a person has successfully quit smoking, he is vulnerable to what we call a relapse for a number of months or perhaps even years. I don't know how many times people attempt to give up smoking but certainly most people who have

quit smoking have had to do it on the second or third try. Your motto should be, 'If I fail, quit and quit again.' "

Announcer: "For a free booklet on quitting smoking, call 1-800-4-CANCER. 1-800-4-CANCER."

The messages were pretested with a group of dedicated smokers to answer the following questions:

1. Does the PSA successfully deliver the major anti-smoking message?
2. Is Dr. Koop perceived to be an appropriate and believable spokesperson for this message?

An intercept technique was used in shopping malls, whereby individuals were shown the PSAs and then asked to respond to a series of questions. Results were very encouraging. Ninety-eight percent of the respondents recognized the message that smoking is hazardous to your health. Another 50 percent indicated that they got the message that smoking causes cancer. Dr. Koop was judged to be a "very appropriate spokesperson" by 72 percent and the messages "very believable" by 70 percent.

Before releasing the spots, television public service directors were asked to evaluate the spots. Both local stations and national networks were shown the PSAs in one-on-one meetings with representatives from OSH, the CIS, and the advertising agency that produced the spots. ABC, NBC, and CBS all granted immediate clearance and the PSAs were enthusiastically received by public service managers. Each network agreed to run the spots in conjunction with appropriate programming.

Advertising agency representatives and regional CIS coordinators distributed the PSAs personally to PSA Directors in 17 major markets. In addition, PSAs were mailed to 900 other television stations throughout the country. Radio PSAs using live announcer copy also were sent out.

Impact of the campaign

Use of the PSAs was measured in several different ways. A Broadcast Advertisers' Report (BAR) survey was contracted, which monitors all television in 75 major markets. Monitoring is done one week each month and figures are projected for the entire month. The PSAs were released in May and June, 1983. As Figure 8.2 shows, airing of the spots rose from 99 times in June to 569 times in July and then slowly declined. Total number of PSAs aired was projected at 1,452 for those months.

Using the estimated number of times the spots were aired, it is pos-

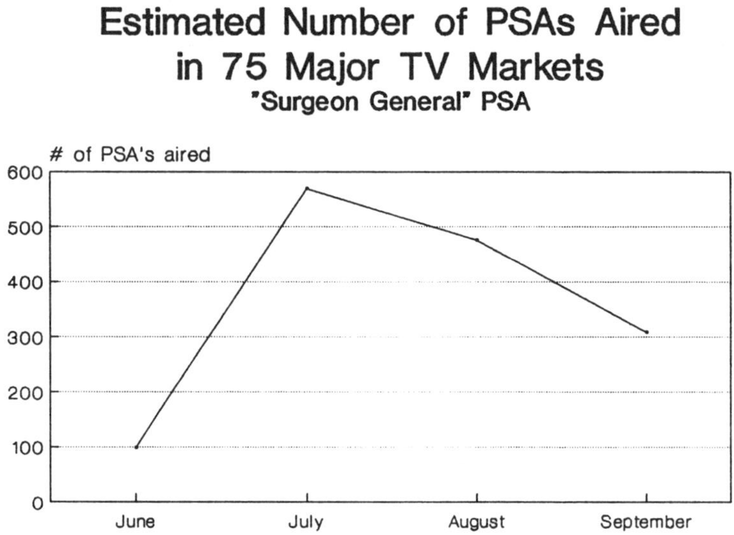

Figure 8.2

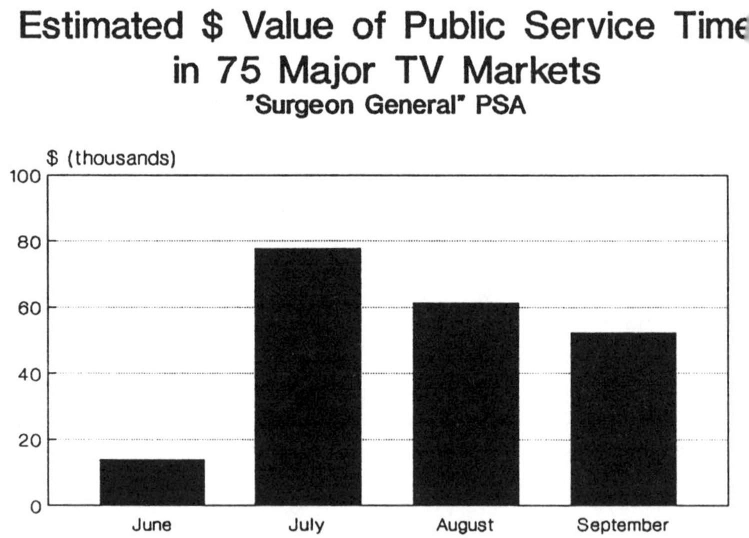

Figure 8.3

Impact of "Surgeon General" PSA on CIS Calls

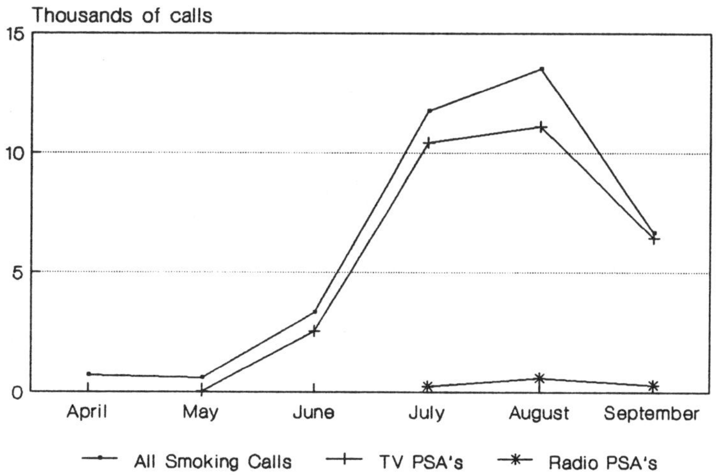

Figure 8.4

sible to calculate the approximate dollar value of the air time given to them based on commercial rates for the market. As noted in Figure 8.3, the dollar value peaked in July and then slowly decreased. The total dollar value of PSA time for these markets was estimated at $205,345, a relatively high figure. These PSAs had a substantial impact on the viewing public. Figure 8.4 illustrates the numbers of calls on smoking received by CIS offices before and during the "Surgeon General" campaign. During April and May, the control months, an average of 600 smoking-related calls per month were received by all CIS offices. By August, during the campaign, calls were up to 13,500 with over 11,000 attributed directly to the PSAs. Over 30,000 calls were stimulated by the PSAs from June through September. Figures 8.2 and 8.4 show that the number of calls to the CIS from the campaign peaked in August, yet the number of spots aired peaked in July. This delay in action supports the belief that several viewings of a PSA are necesssary in order to motivate action.

The third line on the graph reflects calls resulting from the radio PSAs. It is obvious that, in this campaign, this medium was not nearly as effective as television in stimulating public interest.

GOOD NEWS: CANCER PREVENTION

"ARETHA FRANKLIN/PROGRESS"

Public Service Announcement—: 30 Color

For Release May 1985 National Cancer Institute

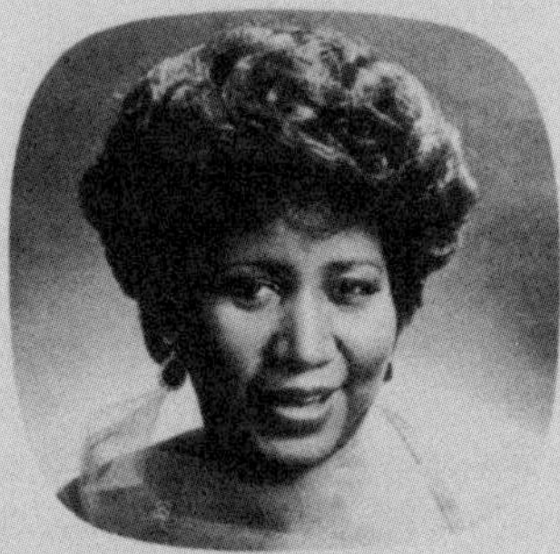

VIDEO	AUDIO
OPEN ON ARETHA FRANKLIN IN HER DRESSING ROOM. CLOSE-UP ON HER THROUGHOUT.	**ANNCR:** Aretha Franklin for the National Cancer Institute!
	ARETHA: (SINGS SCAT) Sha-ba-do-be-do-dwee-dow . . .
	MUSIC UNDER AND THROUGHOUT.
SUPER: ARETHA FRANKLIN.	**ARETHA:** There's a high note in all this talk about cancer: progress in research is giving Blacks hope!
SUPER: CANCER INFORMATION SERVICE. CALL TOLL-FREE 1-800-4-CANCER.	To find out more, call for your cancer prevention booklet. It's free from the Cancer Information Service. Call toll-free, 1-800-4-CANCER.
	When you see how good your chances are against cancer . . .
	MUSIC UP.
	ARETHA: (SING OUT) . . . you'll be on a high note, too! Sha-ba-do-be-do-dwee-dow!

NCI
National Cancer Institute

Figure 8.5

This series of PSAs was successful. The messages were timely; the spokesperson was believable; the public had a place to call for materials and information and they did so.

Aretha Franklin PSA

Campaign development

Motivated by strong evidence that cancer is associated with personal behavior choices and that the public's view of cancer is confused and skeptical, NCI developed the National Cancer Prevention Awareness program which was publicly launched in early 1984. Black Americans are a critical target audience for this program since for many forms of cancer, cancer incidence and mortality rates are higher for blacks than for whites. Specifically, black Americans are at a higher than average risk for cancer of the lung, larynx, throat, respiratory tract, bladder, kidney, and pancreas.

Description of the campaign materials

This campaign included print media kits, press releases, videotapes, and PSAs. In addition, NCI collaborated with leaders in the black community such as historically black colleges, universities, and churches, and the National Association for the Advancement of Colored People to stimulate community involvement.

Following two waves of cancer prevention PSAs targeted to the general public, in June 1985, NCI distributed 450 copies of two television PSAs developed by the Michigan CIS, featuring Aretha Franklin, a well-known black singer, as the spokesperson. These PSAs were targeted specifically toward blacks and were distributed to stations in the top 50 television markets in the United States. Each PSA included a tag at the end containing the telephone number of the CIS to call for more information. (See Figure 8.5.)

Impact of the campaign

Each PSA package contained a postage-paid postcard containing a brief questionnaire on which public service directors could predict their airing of the PSAs. An analysis of the bounceback cards from the Aretha Franklin PSAs shows that of those stations returning the cards, 90 percent indicated that they would air the PSA an average of five or fewer times per week for an average of about 16 weeks.

An analysis of calls made by blacks to the CIS during the Cancer Prevention Awareness campaign showed a 20-fold increase in calls (15 to

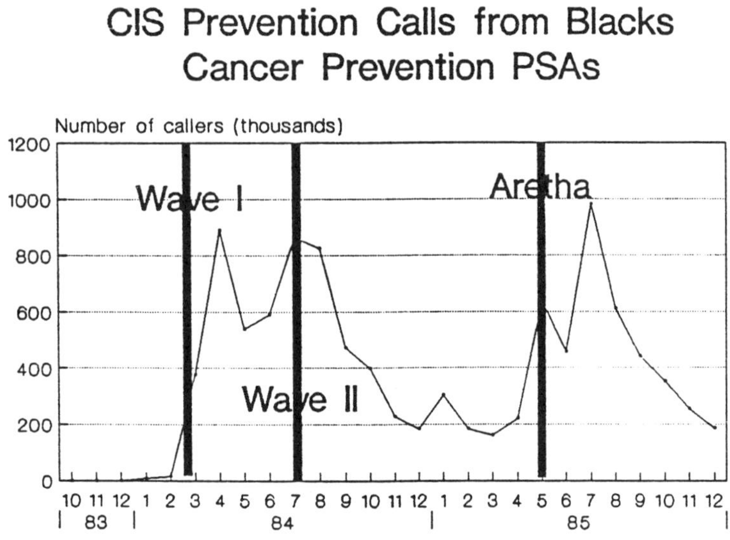

Figure 8.6

378) about cancer prevention after the first wave of general cancer prevention PSAs were distributed. Prevention calls from blacks increased from 589 to 865 after the second wave of general PSAs were aired. More importantly, however, Figure 8.6 shows that prevention calls from blacks almost tripled (222 to 641) following distribution and airing of the specially targeted Aretha Franklin PSAs.

Another way of examining the impact of targeting messages to black audiences is to calculate the percentage of all prevention calls that are made by blacks and see if that proportion changes after a targeted PSA campaign. From October 1983 to May 1985 (prior to the Aretha Franklin PSAs), prevention calls from blacks consistently represented between four and seven percent of the total prevention calls. Following the Aretha Franklin PSAs, the percentage of prevention calls from blacks increased to between 10 and 16 percent. Obviously, PSAs targeted specifically to blacks were followed by disproportionately high responses from blacks.

Additionally, all CIS callers are asked to identify their first source of knowledge of the CIS. An analysis of these answers shows that for the six months after the Aretha Franklin PSAs, 3,196 callers specifically identified the "Aretha" PSA as their source of information about the CIS. Of these 3,196 calls, blacks accounted for 2,767 or 86 percent. Clearly, the strategy of targeting cancer prevention messages directly to the black audience was successful.

Kellogg/NCI Collaboration

Campaign development

One of the specific recommendations from NCI's Cancer Prevention Awareness campaign—eat high fiber food—prompted the Kellogg Company, a large U.S. cereal manufacturer, to request a meeting with NCI to discuss ways of helping NCI disseminate this important message. In June 1984, Kellogg proposed developing print and broadcast advertisements for their All-Bran cereal that would contain an abbreviated version of NCI's dietary message. In addition, Kellogg proposed to summarize the full NCI dietary message on the back panel of the All-Bran cereal box. Kellogg would also include the CIS number, 1-800-4-CANCER, in all advertisements and labeling.

Kellogg introduced the new advertising campaign on October 7, 1984. This collaborative effort between a government agency and a profit-making corporation is an innovative promotion approach.

Description of the campaign materials

The advertising focused on the relationship of a high fiber, low fat diet with reduction of cancer risk and emphasized the fact that Kellogg's All-Bran is a high fiber food. The ads specifically stated that NCI recommends a diet high in fiber and low in fat because it "may reduce the risk of some types of cancer." The campaign was developed by the J. Walter Thompson advertising agency. The first round of advertising introducing the campaign included full page ads in major Sunday newspapers and weekly magazines. The print ads highlighted the information linking diet and cancer risk and listed an address to write for a free booklet on cancer prevention.

The first three 30-second TV spots have been described as "low-key and thoughtful" (Wolinsky, 1985, pp. 4–5); PSA-like; and "startlingly intimate" (Matza, 1985). Each spot opened with an extreme close-up of a speaker describing how he or she has changed his or her diet to include bran cereal after reading new reports from the National Cancer Institute. One, called "Anniversary" showed a woman in her mid-thirties twirling her wedding band. "We had our tenth anniversary last week," she said. "It made me think about things like . . . cereal. That sounds silly, but I just read about new reports from the National Cancer Institute. Some studies suggest a high-fiber, low-fat diet may reduce the risk of some kinds of cancer." After picking up a box of All-Bran, she said: "So we made some changes. Like eating this. Kellogg's All-Bran. 'Cause, ounce for ounce, no food has more fiber than All-Bran. Staying healthy. That's something to celebrate."

Another spot featured an athletic looking woman who has also been described as "a bit tired and worried, even a little tense." (Matza, 1985). She ended the commercial by saying, "Am I gonna change what I eat for breakfast? You better believe it."

Matza (1985) called the third spot the most manipulative. A man said "I have three reasons for eating foods like Kellogg's All-Bran," and then unfolded a string of photos that showed a daughter in pigtails, a son in overalls holding a toy airplane, and his wife. Matza (1985) claimed that "The ominous possibility of a premature death hovers all around him as he talks about the NCI studies and the high-fiber advantages of All-Bran."

These TV spots were radical departures from the conventional cereal advertising formula which one industry spokesman described as "have somebody eat it and smile." (Matza, 1985). The ads also represented the first time a commercial product had been linked with one of America's most dreaded diseases—cancer. In fact, some marketers have called this strategy "bold, innovative, risky and gutsy."(Neiman, 1984, pp. 6–7). Not all reactions were so positive. Lippert (1984) reported that some believed the ads "trivialize the enormity of the disease and grossly inflate the benefits of this product."(p. 40). For others, the issue was a moral one: "Should marketers trade off the fear of cancer as a way to build brand share?"(Lippert, 1984, p. 40).

In mid 1985, Kellogg introduced a second round of TV ads for All-Bran consisting of three new 30-second commercials which followed the same message approach as the original commercials. Late in 1985, a single 30-second commercial was released to introduce All-Bran with Extra Fiber, a new cereal which has the highest fiber content of any cereal currently on the market. Levy and Stokes (1987) report that during 1985, Kellogg spent more than $28 million on high fiber cereal advertising, 50 percent of which was devoted to All-Bran advertisements.

The cereal box information highlighted the NCI's full diet messages and listed the CIS toll-free number and an address for readers to obtain a free booklet on cancer prevention (see Figure 8.7). Kellogg devoted the entire back panel of its All-Bran boxes to NCI's health message. Initially, the packaging approach also included several other Kellogg high fiber cereals.

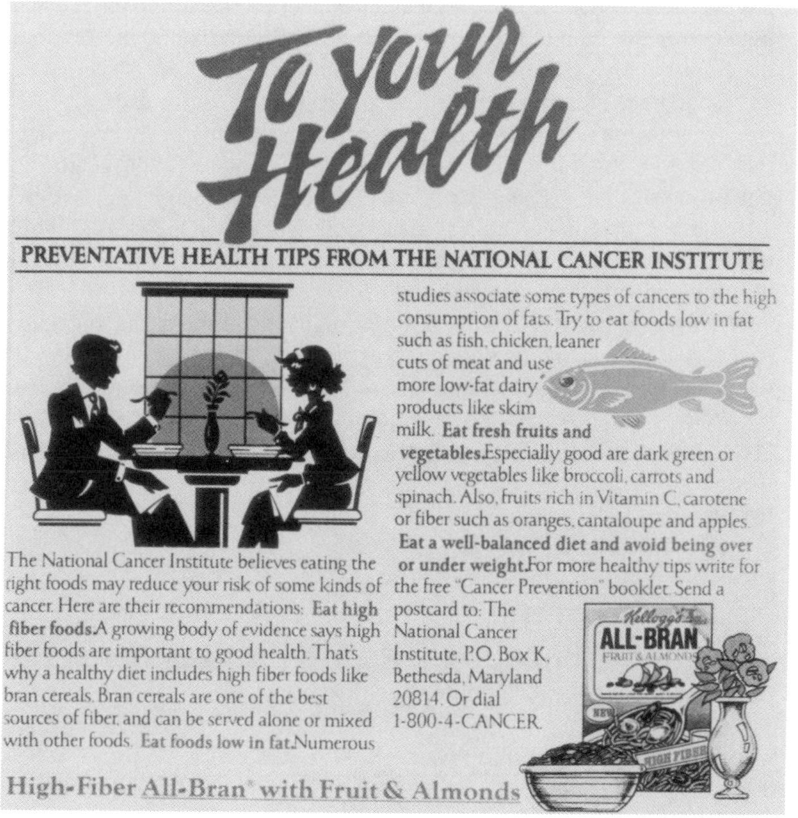
To your Health
PREVENTATIVE HEALTH TIPS FROM THE NATIONAL CANCER INSTITUTE
The National Cancer Institute believes eating the right foods may reduce your risk of some kinds of cancer. Here are their recommendations: **Eat high fiber foods.** A growing body of evidence says high fiber foods are important to good health. That's why a healthy diet includes high fiber foods like bran cereals. Bran cereals are one of the best sources of fiber, and can be served alone or mixed with other foods. **Eat foods low in fat.** Numerous studies associate some types of cancers to the high consumption of fats. Try to eat foods low in fat such as fish, chicken, leaner cuts of meat and use more low-fat dairy products like skim milk. **Eat fresh fruits and vegetables.** Especially good are dark green or yellow vegetables like broccoli, carrots and spinach. Also, fruits rich in Vitamin C, carotene or fiber such as oranges, cantaloupe and apples. **Eat a well-balanced diet and avoid being over or under weight.** For more healthy tips write for the free "Cancer Prevention" booklet. Send a postcard to: The National Cancer Institute, P.O. Box K, Bethesda, Maryland 20814. Or dial 1-800-4-CANCER.
ALL-BRAN
High-Fiber All-Bran® with Fruit & Almonds

Figure 8.7

Kellogg created a public relations campaign to foster media interest in the importance of fiber and its relationship to health. They contacted approximately 63,000 health professionals with mailings about fiber. In addition, they reached approximately 23 million readers through consumer publications. Kellogg also arranged speaking opportunities at professional meetings throughout 1985 to introduce health professionals to this new information on diet and cancer.

Impact of the campaign

The NCI/Kellogg advertising campaign increased consumer knowledge, attitudes, and practices regarding nutrition and dietary habits, especially as they relate to fiber. In a 1985 survey conducted by NCI and the Food and Drug Administration (FDA), nearly one-half of the general public said they had heard or read about cancer prevention in the preceeding six months. In addition, a survey conducted in 1986 by the FDA and the National Heart, Lung, and Blood Institute found that 32 percent of its respondents identified eating fiber as a preventative for cancer.

This increase in knowledge of the health benefits of fiber has naturally led to a jump in cereal sales. *Consumer Reports* (1986) states that All-Bran sales have soared 41 percent since the campaign began. Obviously, other food manufacturers are anxious to share in the wealth, which has recently prompted proposed revisions in federal regulations covering health claims in advertisements and package labeling.

This campaign provided an opportunity to monitor the impact of purchased media time and space as opposed to the usual public service time, on calls to the CIS offices. From November 1984 through December 1986, 13,653 people reported calling specifically in response to the cereal boxes, and 10,650 people called in response to the televised commercials. Figure 8.8 illustrates the trend in calls over the two years monitored.

The cereal boxes with the NCI message and the CIS telephone num-

Impact of Kellogg's Campaign on CIS Calls

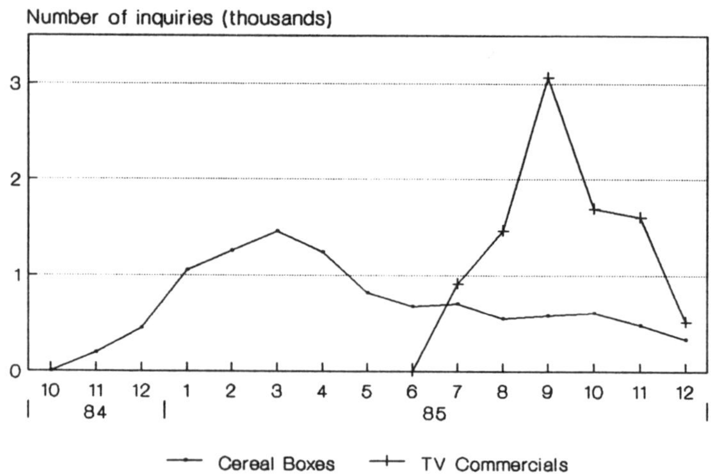

Figure 8.8

ber were placed on grocery store shelves in November 1984, and the commericals featuring the CIS telephone number first aired from July 22-August 12, 1985. As the figure illustrates, calls generated by the cereal boxes began in November 1984, and after a modest peak several months later, continued at a steady pace throughout the time period illustrated. In contrast, the television commercials generated a response that sharply peaked during the time of airing and took three months to decline fully.

All of these studies confirm that the Kellogg campaign had a significant impact on consumers' knowledge, attitudes, and practices regarding fiber in the diet. Consumers seem to be better informed about fiber and its relationship to cancer prevention since the Kellogg campaign. In addition, more consumers indicate eating bran cereals since the campaign began. Although it is not possible to directly attribute these changes to the Kellogg campaign, it seems reasonable to assume the campaign was quite influential. The CIS data provided an opportunity to directly link the campaign to the consumer reaction. Nearly 25,000 calls were made to the CIS in the first two years after the campaign by individuals who specifically identified either the cereal box or the TV commerical as the motivation for their call.

Unplanned Events as Promotion

Less predictable but often more effective in creating a public response are those opportunities that are unexpected but stimulate public interest in a health issue. Most of this unplanned publicity has involved famous people who have been diagnosed as having cancer or who have died of the disease. Betty Ford's, Happy Rockfeller's, and Nancy Reagan's mastectomies prompted thousands of women to get breast examinations and mammograms. John Wayne's fight against lung cancer increased the public's awareness of that disease. A recent example, President Reagan's colon cancer will be discussed in detail later in this section. Ellen Goodman, the newspaper columnist, calls this phenomenon, "the rotating star system, the disease-of-the-month club" (Goodman, 1985, p. A19).

The influence of this "rotating star system" is demonstrated in three studies of newspaper coverage of cancer done in 1977, 1980, and 1984 (Freimuth, Greenberg, DeWitt, and Romano, 1984; Macro Systems, 1986). In 1977 the topic, famous people and cancer, accounted for 26 percent of the 2,138 cancer news stories analyzed and was the second most frequent major topic of these cancer news stories. In 1980, these stories about famous people and cancer accounted for 16 percent of 1,466 cancer news stories analyzed and again was the second most frequent major topic. However, in 1984, there were no famous people being treated for or dying from cancer, and the total number of stories from the same number of days sampled dropped to 796.

These stories about famous people suffering from diseases apparently can educate the public. President Eisenhower suffered a heart attack in 1955 in the middle of a study tracking the public's knowledge of coronary thrombosis over time (Pratt, 1956). Before the President's illness, 38 percent of the respondents knew about coronary thrombosis; after the heart attack and the media publicity surrounding it, 59 percent of the respondents knew about the disease. Pratt summarized the results of this study;

> This difference of 21 percentage points suggests that a significant gain in knowledge resulted from the dissemination of information in connection with the President's illness." (p. 33).

In the two examples that follow, President Reagan's colon cancer and the announcement of a new treatment for cancer, CIS staff at NCI and regional offices made a concerted effort to inform the media of the existence of the CIS and the fact that it was available as an information resource. Without these efforts immediately following the announcements, the impact on the CIS would probably have been negligible.

President Reagan's Colon Cancer

President Reagan's surgery in 1985 for colon cancer provided an opportunity to examine the effect of this kind of unplanned promotion on the public's use of the CIS. Before July 1986, cancer communicators had experienced little success in getting media coverage of colon/rectum cancer. The studies of newspaper coverage of cancer in 1977, 1980, and 1984 provide evidence of this failure (Freimuth, et al., 1984; Macro Systems, 1986). Colon/rectum cancer, which had the highest actual incidence rate in 1977 and the second highest rate in 1980 and 1984, ranked seventh in terms of frequency of news items in 1977, sixth in 1980, and eighth in 1984. In fact, officials of the American Cancer Society had even met with reporters from major newspapers prior to the summer of 1985 to ask how to get coverage of colon/rectum cancer. An ACS official concluded after this meeting, "The only way to break this story was if it happened to a well-known person." (Landis, 1985, p. 42).

This prediction certainly proved accurate when President Reagan's colon cancer was announced on July 15, 1985. National newspapers and magazines ran diagrams of intestines, showed pictures of colonoscopes, and freely used words like "rectum" and "stool." A public who may never have heard or seen mention of the colon or rectum in the mass media before this announcement could tell you the difference between a Dukes A and a Dukes C tumor (terms used to identify the extent of the disease present) as a result of this extensive media coverage.

Impact on the CIS

All of this media attention to colon/rectum cancer dramatically affected the use of the CIS. Before the announcement of Reagan's cancer, the CIS received about 50 calls about colon/rectum cancer per day. For the few days immediately after Reagan's surgery that number jumped to 1,250 calls per day. (See Figure 8.9 for newspaper headlines reflecting the public's response.) As Figure 8.10 shows, even after the initial influx of calls receded, the number of calls did not drop to the previous level.

We contrasted the calls asking about colon/rectum cancer for the six months prior to Reagan's cancer surgery with those calls from the 20 days following the surgery. The calls stimulated by this unplanned publicity were quite different from the usual calls asking about colon/rectum cancer. First, before the Reagan publicity, most calls about colon/rectum cancer came from cancer patients and family/friends of cancer patients (59.1%); however, during the publicity following Reagan's surgery, most of the calls about colon/rectum cancer came from the general public (68.9%). Curiously, the publicity surrounding Reagan's cancer did not seem to increase the number of calls about colon/rectum cancer coming from symptomatic persons. About 15 percent of all colon/rectum calls both before and after Reagan's surgery came from symptomatic people or family/friends of symptomatic people.

This publicity did seem to stimulate people to call the CIS who had never done so before. Before Reagan's surgery, 75.8 percent of the callers who asked about colon/rectum cancer were first time users of the system. Following Reagan's surgery, however, 90.9 percent of the callers were using the system for the first time. As might be expected, the callers who used the system after the publicity surrounding Reagan's cancer reported having learned about the CIS from television and newspapers much more frequently than the previous callers asking about colon/rectum cancer.

The focus on President Reagan in the publicity seemed to serve to target the information especially to older males. Following Reagan's sur-

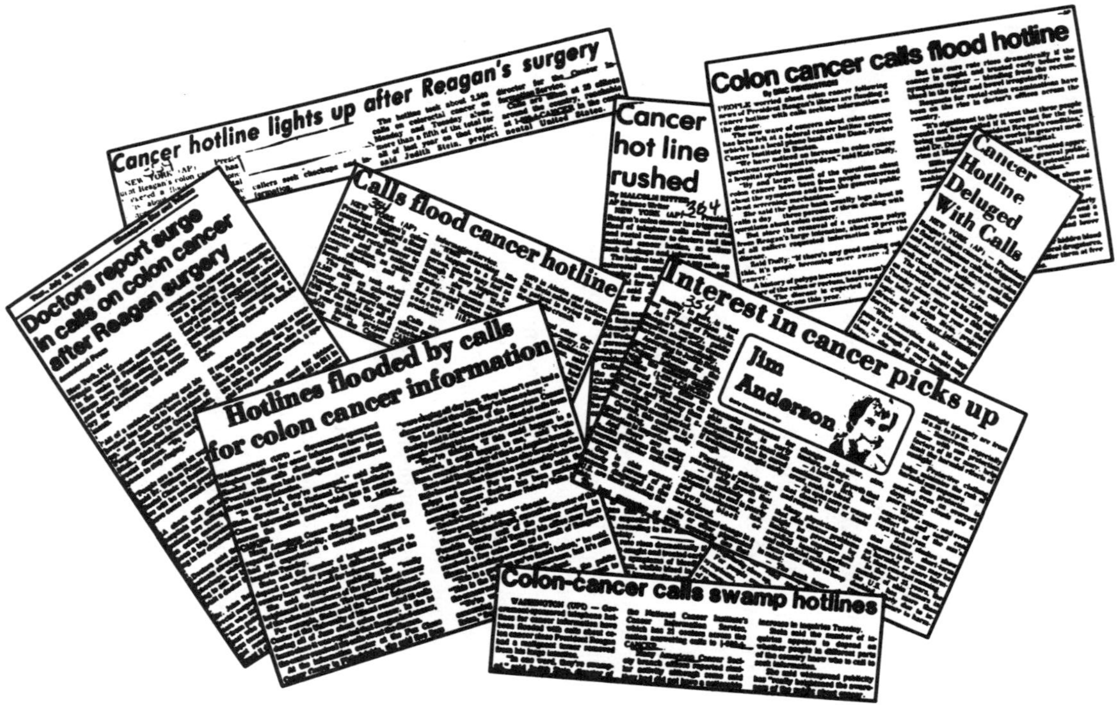
Cancer hotline lights up after Reagan's surgery
Cancer hot line rushed
Colon cancer calls flood hotline
Cancer Hotline Deluged With Calls
Doctors report surge in calls on colon cancer after Reagan surgery
Calls flood cancer hotline
Interest in cancer picks up
Jim Anderson
Hotlines flooded by calls for colon cancer information
Colon-cancer calls swamp hotlines

Figure 8.9

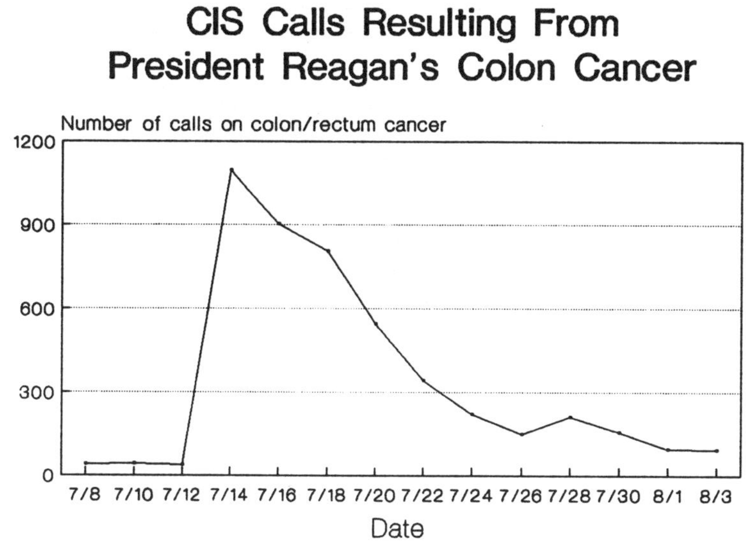

Figure 8.10

gery, 38.8 percent of the calls asking about colon/rectum cancer came from males compared to only 29.8 percent prior to Reagan's cancer. The same effect was observed for age. Prior to the publicity about Reagan's cancer, 23.5 percent of all calls asking about colon/rectum cancer came from callers aged 60 or older, but, after the publicity started, 38.4 percent of these calls came from these older callers. The publicity did not seem to affect the education or ethnic distributions of callers.

The subjects inquired about in these calls were quite different before and after this publicity. As Figure 8.11 shows, the individuals calling before Reagan's surgery asked mostly about general cancer information, treatment, and local organizations and services. After Reagan's surgery, however, most callers inquired about general cancer information or prevention.

The system responded to these colon/rectum calls differently before and after the publicity. Although the same three behavioral suggestions were given most often, the frequency was quite different before and after the publicity. (See Figure 8.12.)

Moreover, the time spent with the caller on the phone was also shorter for those who called after Reagan's surgery; three-fourths of these

Subject of Inquiry for Calls Placed Before and After Reagan's Surgery
Cancer Information Service, 1983-86

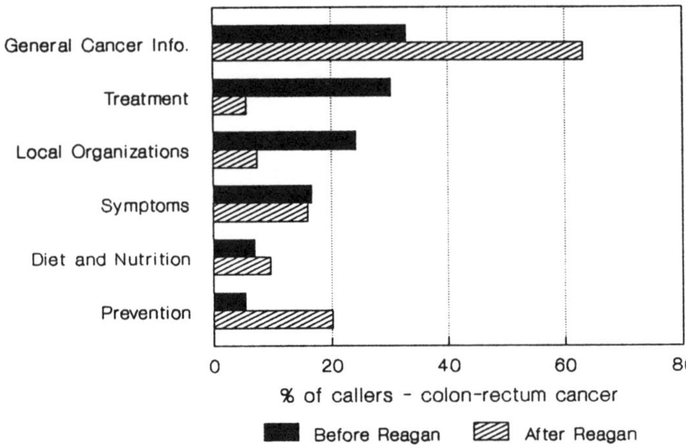

Figure 8.11

Behavioral Suggestions Given Before and After Reagan's Surgery
Cancer Information Service, 1983-86

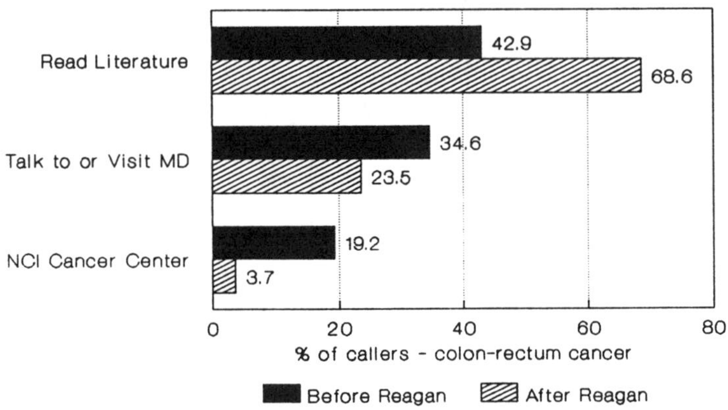

Figure 8.12

calls were five minutes or less whereas only half of the colon/rectum calls made before Reagan's surgery were this short. Considering both the preponderance of suggestions to read the literature and the brevity of most of these calls stimulated by the publicity surrounding Reagan's cancer, we question whether the CIS took full advantage of its opportunity to influence the new information seeker who was keenly interested in colon/rectum cancer when he/she made the call. The CIS might have lost an opportunity to encourage some beneficial changes in health behavior. On the other hand, the brevity of the calls may well have been due to the large number of calls handled during a relatively short time period, putting pressure on the CIS staff to turn to the next caller. Fast breaking events which generate surges in incoming calls are an inherent problem in a system such as the CIS where staffing and numbers of incoming lines remain relatively constant.

This comparison of the calls before and after the unplanned publicity surrounding President Reagan's cancer demonstrates the opportunities created by this kind of event. Not only did the number of calls about this heretofore "unmentionable" cancer increase enormously, but the profile of the callers broadened from primarily cancer patients asking about treatment and services to the general public interested in prevention, many of whom were new users of the CIS. Reaching this group of people created a prevention opportunity that may not have been exploited as well as it should have been. Although the national and regional offices did an excellent job of working with the press to insure that their phone number would be included in information about this publicity, perhaps the constraints of limited phone lines and staff prevented them to some extent from capitalizing on the information seeking which did result.

Interleukin-2

The second example of unplanned publicity was the news of the discovery of a new treatment for cancer. The public's expectations rise every time there is any news that a scientific breakthrough may have occurred in the search for a cure for cancer. Therefore, the NCI moved cautiously in announcing early findings on the LAK cell/interleukin-2 therapy developed and tested in its laboratories and clinics. A major problem for NCI had been to decide when to publish preliminary clinical data (DeVita, 1986). Early steps in the research had been reported at scientific meetings and scientists were asking for the data. Moreover, NCI wanted to expand the clinical trials to other medical centers but needed to have the data undergo peer review first. The decision was made to publish the data and they appeared in the *New England Journal of Medicine* on December 5, 1985. In fact, NCI was so cautious about raising false hopes that it unveiled the news in a routine "Update" bulletin rather than a press conference.

The media paid more attention to the story than had been expected at NCI. As Paul Van Nevel, Associate Director for Communications at the NCI, said, "We expected it was going to raise a lot of attention based on what was written in the scientific journals. But instead it was just like an explosion." (Richburg, 1985, p. A3). The *Washington Post* and the *Miami Herald* ran the story on the first page but the *New York Times* ran an Associated Press report on page 19. ABC and NBC led their evening news shows with announcement of the treatment and its success.

Impact on the CIS

As a result of all this publicity, the public flooded the CIS with over 1000 inquiries per day about this new treatment. Most of these calls were from families and friends of cancer patients who were desperately looking for hope for their loved ones. One caller told a CIS information specialist,

> "My mother had a malignant brain tumor. The doctor says it will grow back and kill her. She has less than a year to live."

A cancer patient calling for himself said,

> "I have colon cancer, a tumor on my liver. My prognosis was three months. I've passed that already. I saw the research on TV and I wanted to see how to get on the program and what it would cost me."

There was some concern about using the CIS telephone number as a resource following the interleukin-2 announcement because, unfortunately, these callers had to be told that the treatment was experimental and there was no more room in the initial study. Even though people could not be referred to this specific study, the CIS management staff felt that this announcement gave them the opportunity to inform callers about other treatment options and clinical research opportunities that might be appropriate. In fact, 40 percent of these callers were referred to NCI's regional comprehensive cancer centers.

We examined those calls asking about clinical trials or immunotherapy (the general classification of treatment for interleukin-2) placed to the CIS from December 5, 1985 to December 25, 1985. Since 85 percent of these calls came from cancer patients or family and friends of cancer patients, we decided to compare these interleukin-2 calls to only those calls from 1983 through 1986 from cancer patients and family/friends of cancer patients.

In general, the callers asking about the new treatment had similar demographic characteristics to cancer patients and family/friends of cancer patients who call about other subjects. The only demographic difference was that there was a higher proportion of males in this group calling about interleukin-2 (36.1% vs. 24.0%) than in the other group of cancer patient and family/friends callers. The site most frequently asked about for these interleukin-2 callers was lung (23.0%) followed by colon/rectum (14.5%) and breast (10.8%); however, for all cancer patients, family/friends of cancer patients callers, the most frequently asked about site was breast (29.6%) followed by lung (16.5%) and colon/rectum (12.7%).

The source of information about the CIS differed for these interleukin-2 callers. They were more likely to hear about the CIS from the mass media—television (25.2%) and newspapers (14.2%)—than were the total group of cancer patients and family/friends of cancer patients.

Both the Reagan cancer story and the interleukin-2 story are examples of unplanned events that can dramatically publicize a service such as the CIS. These events also reinforce the importance of conceiving of the information service as a comprehensive communication system which must be primed both to stimulate and react to promotion activities.

Summary

A comprehensive communication system such as the CIS must promote itself if it expects to be used. In some cases, that promotion must create uncertainly where it may not already exist in order to stimulate information seeking. In other cases, the promotion needs to create awareness of the information service itself so that those already engaged in an information search will have another resource to consult. The CIS uses planned promotions at the national and regional levels and tries to capitalize on unplanned events for promoting itself. Although many communication channels are used in these efforts, most of the national promotion resources have been devoted to television public service announcements.

When these promotion campaigns are evaluated, it is quite clear that they do have an impact on the number of calls received from various audiences and on the nature of the questions asked. On the other hand, the public's interests affect the CIS as well. If an unplanned event stimulates interest in a particular type of cancer or treatment, the information system must be primed to respond to these demands. Therefore the CIS is a communication system which reflects an interactive model of communication rather than the static, linear model which governs too many information dissemination efforts.

9

Knowledge and Utilization Gaps

In spite of the successful promotion of the CIS, we have seen consistent patterns of underutilization by the minority and less educated members of all three user groups examined. From these data, we cannot tell if these less educated consumers are not engaging in any information searches or are just not using the CIS as one of their information sources. This utilization gap is quite significant because low income and poorly educated individuals and minorities are frequently at higher risk for many health problems, including cancer. Hence, they are the primary targets for numerous health information campaigns. Yet when these same campaigns are evaluated, these groups usually emerge as less exposed, less knowledgeable, and less likely to change their behaviors. In fact, there is some evidence that health communications campaigns actually increase the knowledge and utilization gaps between the information "haves" and "have nots." This chapter explores these gaps by describing the characteristics of the information poor, reviewing theoretical explanations of the utilization and knowledge gaps, and analyzing data from the minority and less educated CIS users.

Characteristics of the Information Poor

This section briefly reviews such characteristics of the information poor as the nature of their subculture, a fatalistic predisposition, limited media usage, and their health information needs.

Nature of the Poverty Subculture

A comprehensive review of literature relating to the information poor was published by Childers and Post in 1975. Apparently no comprehensive update of this literature has been done since. Much of the following information is taken from this 1975 review and the reader must keep in mind that this information is dated. The following list presents the different groups Childers includes in his description of the information poor:

1. Mexican-Americans, Puerto Ricans, and other Spanish speaking people.
2. American Indians and Eskimos.
3. Poor black Americans and whites.
4. Appalachians.
5. Poor farmers.
6. Migrant workers.
7. Aging adults.
8. The blind or deaf.
9. Prisoners.

Economically disadvantaged persons include nearly 34 million Americans, 23 million whites, 9.5 million blacks, and 1.2 million of other races (U.S. Bureau of the Census, 1987). Of these poor, over 3 million are elderly persons 65 years and older and more than one million are migrant agricultural workers.

Information universe of the disadvantaged

Childers and Post (1975) suggest that economically disadvantaged people share some characteristics that affect their information universe. One of the first barriers for these people is the level of processing skills at their command. Reading ability is often quite low. English may be a second language. These disadvantaged people may have little experience in the communication skills we take for granted, such as bargaining for a car or negotiating a contract on a house.

Second, the disadvantaged are often locked into an information ghetto. Their information system is a closed one—any contact from the outside usually comes through the mass media, a one-way flow of information. As a result, much misinformation is prevalent. Internally generated information is accepted and disseminated similarly to other communities. But, as Childers and Post (1975) put it, "there is a kind of social embargo against a great body of externally generated information." (p. 33).

The third major barrier among the disadvantaged is a fatalistic predisposition. Some research on the poor portrays them as despairing, fatalistic people with a pervasive sense of helplessness. Locus of control has been another popular construct used to describe this predisposition. Disadvantaged people are seen as more likely to exhibit an external locus of control, meaning that their lives are controlled by outside forces over which they have little control. Niemi and Anderson (1971) describe this predisposition differently. They speak of a "lower-class value stretch" in which people do not abandon the general values of society but generate an alternative set of values rationalized to fit their status.

The way the disadvantaged use available channels of communication is another barrier. As is the case with the general public, the disadvantaged have access to both informal and formal sources of information and prefer the informal sources to meet specific information needs. When the disadvantaged person does perceive a need for information and seeks it, there is evidence that the search is less intense (Childers and Post, 1975).

The other consistent conclusion in information channels studies is the low level of readership among the disadvantaged. For example, Block (1972) studied mass media exposure patterns of blacks in St. Louis and found that 40 percent did not read at all or less than one hour per week. Yet these same respondents rated newspapers as the most important information source, TV second, friends third, and advice from social workers last. In a public opinion survey of a black ghetto in Pittsburgh in 1967, 72 percent reported reading only a small portion of the newspaper; very few reported using it for news.

Television is always reported as the source most frequently used by the poor. It is unclear, however, whether television is being used for entertainment or for information. Olien, Donohue, and Tichenor (1978) found that as education went up, preferences for newspapers increased and preferences for television went down. Parker and his associates' (1966) explanation for these findings was that education increases the need for information and reduces the need for escape.

Childers and Post (1975) reported a classification of information as either "ends" information or "means" information. The former relates to what one wants to achieve and the latter relates to how to achieve it. The electronic media contain more "ends" information and the print media more "means" information. Childers and Post (1975) described the dilemma created by the overreliance of the disadvantaged adult on the electronic media:

> He is overexposed to "ends" information through television and radio, and sorely underexposed to the kind of information that might help him achieve the ends that he desires. (p. 40).

Childers and Post (1975) summarized their review of the information poor with this portrait of the disadvantaged adult in his/her natural information habitat:

> Does not know which formal channels to tap in order to solve his problems, or what specific programs exist to respond to his needs.
>
> Watches many hours of television daily, seldom reads newspapers and magazines, and never reads books.
>
> Does not see his problems as information needs.
>
> Is not a very active information seeker, even when he does undertake a search.
>
> May lean heavily on formal channels of information if it becomes apparent that the informal channels are inadequate and if his need is strongly felt.
>
> Is locked into an informal information network that is deficient in the information that is ordinarily available to the rest of society. (pp. 42–43).

Health information needs of the disadvantaged

Bergner and Yerby (1968) presented a vivid description of the health status of the poor.

> The poor behave differently from the middle class and the affluent across a wide spectrum related to health care. Illness is defined differently. There is less accurate health information. The poor are less inclined to take preventive measures, and delay longer in seeking medical care. When they do approach health practitioners, they are more likely to select subprofessionals or the marginal practitioners often found in their neighborhoods. (p. 543).

Heagarty, Robertson, Kosa, and Alpert (1968) reinforced this picture by describing the health care of low-income families as fragmented, episodic, and crisis-oriented, and likely to occur in a public clinic or hospital outpatient setting. Some recent statistics confirm the low health status of disadvantaged people. The National Center for Health Statistics

(1987) reported that infant mortality was 10.6 per 1000 births for the total US population and 9.3 for whites, but 18.2 for blacks. Smoking is another health risk that affects the disadvantaged more than the rest of society. Smoking is most common among the less educated and the less successful. Twenty-six percent of men in professional and technical fields smoke while 50 percent of men in blue-collar jobs smoke.

Childers and Post (1975) summarized four major problems related to the health information environment of the disadvantaged adult:

1. They tend to know less about diseases—warning signals, symptoms, communicability.
2. They tend not to know about preventive health services, such as pre-natal care, dental care or health insurance.
3. They tend not to know where to turn for health services in general, and they do not know which specific services are available.
4. Folk-medicine—both the formal kind, like shamanism, and the informal kind, like backwoods herbal pharmacology—is well entrenched among the non-urban disadvantaged. (pp. 44–45).

A special ACS report (1985) found that a person's chances of survival after a diagnosis of cancer have more to do with his or her economic status than with racial or ethnic background. In fact, the report revealed that the 34 million poor have a relative cancer survival rate of 10 to 15 percent below the American overall rate of approximately 50 percent. Baquet and Ringen (1986) include socio-economic status as one of five key factors related to cancer survival. They describe the effects of SES in the following way:

> Socioeconomic status has major ramifications on health resources, including accessibility, availability, utilization, quality, and continuity of health services, including state-of-the-art cancer screening, detection, treatment, and rehabilitation. In addition, SES affects nutritional status and dietary patterns, immune status and function, educational level/attitude and awareness of cancer preventive concepts/behaviors, acceptance of cancer as a real and occupational hazard exposure. Many of these factors accumulate over time and interact to reinforce each other thus enhancing the overall effect. (Baquet and Ringen, 1986, p. 219)

The Knowledge Gap Hypothesis

Historically, studies of mass media effects have demonstrated that education correlates strongly with acquisition of knowledge about public affairs and science from mass media. Tichenor, Donohue, and Olien (1970) formalized this observation in the knowledge gap hypothesis which predicts that as mass media information is infused into a social system, members with more education acquire knowledge faster than do those with relatively less education. Consequently, the gap in knowledge between the two social groups increases rather than decreases. Predictions are made for both one-time and multiple measurements:

> **1.** Over time, acquisition of knowledge of a heavily publicized topic will proceed at a faster rate among better educated persons than among those with less education.
> **2.** At a given point in time, there should be a higher correlation between acquisition of knowledge and education for topics highly publicized in the media than for topics less highly publicized. (Tichenor, et al., 1970, p. 165).

The knowledge gap hypothesis includes three variables: level of mass media publicity in a particular setting, level of individuals' education, and level of individuals' knowledge about a specific subject. Time may be included as a fourth variable. Yet the term "knowledge gap" appearing in the literature may have several different meanings. In Gaziano's (1983) review of over 58 studies of the knowledge gap, she found it important to distinguish among the following meanings of the knowledge gap: (1) gaps found at one point in time; (2) gaps which may occur over time and may change in magnitude; (3) gaps which refer only to the relationship between education and knowledge without reference to media; and (4) gaps which result from media treatment or media exposure. Gaziano concluded from her review that most of the research supported the proposition that the higher the education, the greater the knowledge of various topics. This relationship does not directly support the original knowledge gap hypothesis, however, because the level of mass media publicity for topics is not considered. Gaziano's conclusion from time-trend studies actually reversed the original knowledge gap hypothesis. She concluded that increasing levels of media publicity may reduce gaps, but that several other factors may be equally or more influential in doing so. Additional evidence refuting the knowledge gap comes from one-time case studies where the frequent finding of moderately sized gaps may indicate that media publicity played a part in decreasing initially larger gaps.

Gaziano (1983) analyzed several varying characteristics of the 58 studies to determine what other variables might have affected the knowledge gap. She found that the most frequent characteristics associated with knowledge inequalities seem to be the type and geographic scope of the topic studied. Gaps are more likely to occur when (1) topics are international and national issues; (2) topics are of greater interest to high socioeconomic status (SES) persons than to low SES individuals; and (3) knowledge is conceptualized in civics class or textbook terms. Gaps occur less often or are smaller when topics are local and are likely to appeal to lower SES strata. There is only limited evidence to help us decide whether health topics and specifically cancer fit this pattern.

Knowledge Gaps in Health

Several studies support the existence of gaps in health knowledge at one point in time. Gaziano (1983) identified several knowledge gap studies of health topics and found that, although people of all educational backgrounds tend to be highly interested in health matters, they may still show knowledge disparities. Butler and Paisley (1976) also argued that health knowledge is unequally distributed throughout society, pointing out that health knowledge "haves" are young, white, and better educated while the "have nots" are old, nonwhite and less educated. Stojanovic's (1972) study of the awareness of Medicare supported this racial difference in knowledge. He found that the proportion of respondents who were unaware of the program was four times as great for blacks than for whites. In their study of the Minnesota Heart Health Program, Lee, Kline, Jacobs, and Hannan (1985) examined individual, family, and community antecedents to health knowledge, and found that educational attainment and involvement in health were the most significant predictors of health knowledge.

Greater education and its correlates of high income and youth also have been found to be associated with knowledge about different aspects of cancer. In a 1977 household survey conducted as part of the Los Angeles Health Survey, scores from 25 questions were added together to produce a general cancer knowledge level score (Stone and Siegel, 1986). This general cancer knowledge index correlated positively with both education ($r = .27$) and income ($r = .13$). When education was used as a predictor variable in a regression analysis of this cancer knowledge index, it entered the regression equation first and income did not enter the equation at all, demonstrating that more of the variance in cancer knowledge could be explained by education than by income. This study also supported the influence of ethnicity on cancer knowledge. Even after controlling for education, behavior, and cancer worry, Hispanics and blacks had significantly lower levels of knowledge than whites, Asians, and others.

A 1978 ACS survey of public attitudes toward cancer and cancer tests provided further evidence of this knowledge gap (Public attitudes toward cancer . . . , 1980). When asked in this survey if they had heard of breast reconstruction, 63 percent of the college-educated women said yes, compared to 47 percent of the high school graduates, and 22 percent of the grade school educated. The most recent evidence of this knowledge gap comes from the NCI's Cancer Prevention Awareness surveys done in two waves, the first one in June, 1983 and the second from February through April, 1985. These surveys discovered that correct or desired responses to "cancer attitude statements" generally increased with education. For example, when asked to respond to the statement, "It seems like everything causes cancer," more respondents disagreed as the educational level increased. In addition, educational attainment served as a good predictor of knowledge of cancer prevention. When asked to react to the statement, "There is not much a person can do to prevent cancer," 39 percent of those who did not attend high school responded correctly; whereas, 66.7 percent of those who graduated from college responded correctly.

There is less consistency with previous research on the way media publicity may affect gaps. Tichenor and his associates (1970) supported the original knowledge gap hypothesis with their 1968 research in two Minnesota cities, measuring recall of medical, biological, and social science topics in the news, and comparing recall to previous amount of newspaper publicity given to these subjects. On the other hand, Ettema, Brown, and Luepker (1983) failed to support the original knowledge gap hypothesis but did support Gaziano's conclusion that media publicity played a part in decreasing initially larger gaps. In their study of the effects of an informational campaign on cardiovascular health, Ettema and his associates found that the campaign virtually eliminated the existing gap between more and less well-educated segments. They identified motivation as a significant factor mediating gap effects.

Based on limited research in the health area, it seems reasonable to conclude that, at any one time, there usually is a gap in the levels of knowledge about most health topics but that increasing the mass media information disseminated about that topic may reduce the gap.

Explanations of the Knowledge Gap

Several alternative explanations have been suggested for the knowledge gap phenomonen. These explanations can be grouped under three categories: those that attribute the knowledge gap to characteristics of the audience, the message, and the social system.

Audience characteristics

Tichenor and his colleagues' (1970) approach to causation is consistent with what other authors have called the individual blame bias (e.g., Rogers, 1983). They suggest that the "information haves" can be described as having:

1. Superior communication skills such as reading and comprehension.
2. Greater stored information increasing awareness and capacity to understand new information.
3. More relevant social contacts who are likely to discuss the issues.
4. Selective exposure, acceptance, and retention to messages which follow from these previous differences.

These audience factors need to be examined in light of what Ettema and Kline (1977) described as the difference versus the deficit thesis. The deficit thesis arose from research examining the achievement gap which assumed that the relationship between SES and intellectual performance was caused by a deficiency of basic cognitive ability. On the other hand, the difference thesis argues that people from different social strata have the same underlying competence as those in the mainstream of the dominant culture, "difference in performance being accounted for by the situations and contexts in which the competence is expressed." (Ettema and Kline, 1977, p. 186). An emphasis on deficits such as lack of communication skills to explain the knowledge gap predicts that gaps will always widen and never narrow. By contrast, the difference thesis predicts that:

> gaps widen in those circumstances in which lower SES persons are less motivated to acquire the information or in which the

> information is less functional for them, while gaps may narrow (and perhaps even fail to materialize in the first place) when the motivation to acquire the information is increased among the lower SES persons or when the information is functional for them. (Ettema and Kline, 1977, p. 188).

Ettema, Brown, and Luepker (1983) believe that interest or motivation rather than education is the key mediating factor in the knowledge gap. Genova and Greenberg (1979) also found composite interest (a combination of social and self interest) to be a better predictor of knowledge than education.

In a later study, Ettema (1984) further supported his argument for interest or motivation outweighing SES as an antecedent of information gain. He found that innovativeness and ability to see the importance of information was more important than SES. The ability to see the importance of information was positively related to system use while family income was negatively related. Moreover, use itself was most strongly related to reported benefits. Dervin (1980) also supports the difference perspective on audience factors when she challenges the construct validity of the knowledge gap because of its underlying traditional model of source-receiver. She favors instead the relativist model which underlies information-seeking and uses and gratifications. Finally, there is the perspective promoted by McKnight (1985), which argues that the problem with lack of knowledge and utilization stems not from lack of information but from a mistrust and even a deliberate rejection of the "establishment" position.

In summary, audience causal factors can be grouped under those consistent with a deficit or a difference perspective. The difference perspective is more useful because it suggests opportunities to narrow or eliminate gaps. The necessary strategy appears to be making the information interesting and functional as well as credible for the specific audience.

Message characteristics

Message characteristics affecting the knowledge gap have usually been discussed as some type of ceiling or upper limits in the knowledge to be disseminated. Ettema and Kline (1977) identified three types of ceilings which often appear in the literature on the knowledge gap: artifacts, imposed ceilings, and true ceilings. Artifacts refer to those ceilings which are only measurement artifacts which may be responsible for data showing lower SES individuals catching up. Cooke and his associates (1975) cited the "Sesame Street" evaluation as an example of the artifact type of ceiling. These authors claim that the measurements used were more sensitive to pre- to post- test improvements by children who scored lower initially than by children who scored higher on the pretest.

Two types of imposed ceilings were described by Ettema and Kline (1977): those imposed by the message itself and those imposed by the audience on themselves. Those ceilings imposed by the message itself occur when the message is simple and limited, and, since the more informed audience members are likely to already have the information, the message allows the less informed audience members to catch up. There is evidence, for example, that the campaigns with the simple message that smoking is harmful to your health have reached nearly everyone and no significant knowledge gap remains. (This is certainly not to suggest that the behavior change has followed the knowledge gain.) The other category of imposed ceilings includes those imposed by the audience upon themselves. Although this type of ceiling is not mentioned directly in the literature, Ettema and Kline (1977) reinterpreted results from a study of family planning and adolescents: better informed adolescents felt that they had enough information and, thus, were not motivated to seek any more, giving less informed adolescents a chance to catch up.

The final type of ceiling, the true ceiling, occurs when the knowledge being disseminated has a definite boundary. Once the "early knowers" have reached this boundary, there is an opportunity for the "later knowers" to catch up. Dramatic news events, such as the assassination of a public figure, are often given as examples of these true ceilings.

When there is a source-imposed ceiling or a true ceiling, gaps should narrow. Similarly, gaps will narrow when the higher SES audience members impose a ceiling on themselves and the lower SES members do not.

Message ceilings already are widely used in the health field to reduce knowledge gaps. Health communicators often develop campaign objectives with a type of ceiling imposed, to reduce the complexity of the desired behavior to its simplest form, e.g., "Don't smoke. Smoking is harmful to your health." and "Wear seat belts. They may save your life."

Social system characteristics

Social system causal factors reflect the shift from individual blame to social system blame. Attributing gaps to the social system rather than the individual also reinforces the appropriateness of the difference thesis over the deficit thesis. Several authors (e.g., Olien, Tichenor, and Donohue, 1982; Tichenor, Donohue, and Olien, 1980) contend that structural variables must be considered, i.e., that the most important knowledge sources were more accessible to the most educated people. For example, these authors argued that it is the nature of the media that most science and public interest information is carried by print, which is more available to high status people.

Ettema (1984) outlined places in the social system where gaps can develop:

1. *Development of the system.* Systems are often created and made available to specialized users who are already information rich (e.g., videotext users, personal health information systems). The development of systems has often been left up to the private sector to determine who will have access and that generally is the higher SES groups. This problem is less significant in the health area because many information systems are developed by the public rather than the private sector.

2. *Adoption of the system.* Adopters tend to be relatively young and better educated, and have an ability to see the information value of the system. Moreover, the desire to adopt the system may reflect less of a need for the information than a desire for it.

The CIS avoids most of these social system problems because the service is free and accessible to anyone with a telephone. However, use of the CIS does require a certain level of communication skills and a recognition of the telephone as a potential information-seeking instrument.

Evidence of the Knowledge Gap in the CIS Data

In order to further investigate the validity of the knowledge gap hypothesis in the area of cancer information, we analyzed the CIS call record form data focusing on the education of CIS callers, dividing them into three groups: (1) those who had only a grade school education but were older than 19 (N = 7,987); (2) those who had some high school and were older than 19 (N = 33,629); and (3) those who were at least high school graduates (N = 1,008,007). These two lower education groups were sometimes further collapsed into a single category for the analysis in this chapter. Although education is only one component of socio-economic status, it correlates strongly with income, is the one indicator most commonly used in research, and is the only one available in this data set.

Comparison of Demographic Characteristics

Educational level did not seem to affect the rate at which men and women used the CIS. Regardless of education, women called the system three times as frequently as men. There was, however, a major difference in age distribution for callers of different educational levels. Almost two-thirds (64.7%) of those callers with only a grade school education were over 50 years while only one-third of those who were at least high school graduates fell into this age range. Clearly for the callers to the CIS, there is a strong inverse relationship between age and education.

Education and ethnicity also were strongly related. Asian and white callers were better educated than black and Hispanic callers. Figure 9.1 shows the proportion of callers from each ethnic group who had grade school and some high school education. Hispanics had the least education of any of the ethnic groups with 16.6 percent of them having less than a high school education. It should be remembered that these percentages do not include those under 19 years of age; therefore, these low

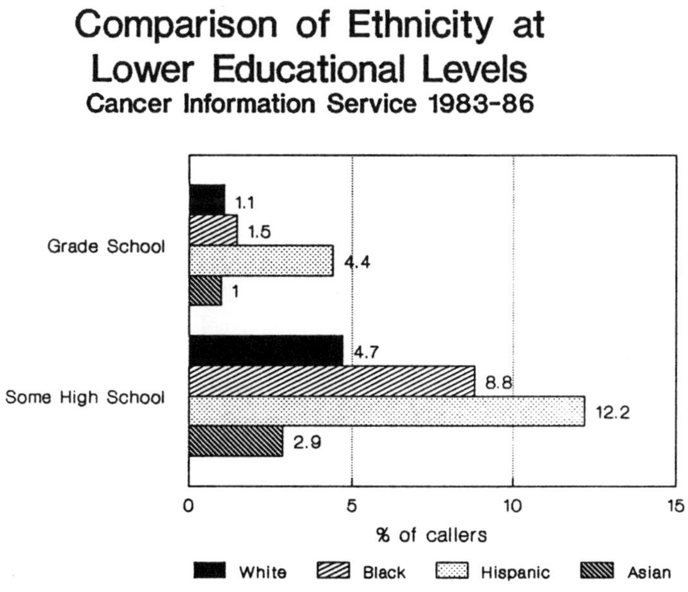

Figure 9.1

educational levels do not just reflect the relative youth of the Hispanic population.

Educational level definitely affects use of the CIS. While 20 percent of callers with at least a high school diploma reported having used the CIS before, only two percent of those callers with less than a high school diploma reported prior experience with the CIS. Clearly this disparity points to at least a utilization gap if not a knowledge gap.

Nature of the Inquiries

There are even some differences in the topics inquired about by callers with different educational levels. The less educated callers are more likely to ask about smoking and other risk factors (31.1% vs. 23.8%) while the more educated callers ask more often about treatment (16.4% vs. 9.2%). The relationship between smoking inquiries and education is not surprising since smoking is more prevalent among less educated people. The number of inquiries about breast and colon/rectum cancers also varied with education. Those with only a grade school education asked less often about breast cancer (29.3% vs. 34.8%) and more often about colon/rectum cancer (22.3% vs. 14.4%) than do those callers who have attained at least a high school education. As we suggested in an earlier chapter, perhaps gastro-intestinal symptoms are less understood by less educated groups and stimulate more uncertainty, prompting calls to the CIS. On the other hand, more educated people may already be more aware of the many treatment options facing breast cancer patients and be calling to further explore these options.

This analysis by education confirmed the trend we had been observing in all our previous data, i.e., the less educated callers rely more on television as a source of information about the CIS (43%) than do the more educated callers (33.4%). The only other difference between the educational levels is that less educated callers also use the ACS as an information source less frequently (4.5%) than do the more educated callers (7.2%).

Responses to Calls

Even though educational level of the caller is not asked until the end of the telephone conversation, it does seem to affect the system's response to the call. For example, the less educated callers are more frequently told to try to quit smoking (19.6% vs. 10.8%), to read literature (56.1% vs. 49.2%) but less frequently referred to a specialized cancer center (5.9% vs. 11.9%). The less educated callers more often receive some type of follow-up to their call (77.9% vs. 67%), usually in the form of publications (74.7%). Perhaps these callers are less informed about cancer and, therefore, their needs are more likely to be satisfied with a general publication.

Since the literature on the knowledge gap often fails to distinguish clearly between low SES and ethnicity, we looked at the educational levels of our callers separately for each of three ethnic groups: blacks, Hispanics, and Asians.

Black Callers

Most of the general demographic differences described above for educational levels were replicated for the black callers. Educational levels did not affect the 3:1 ratio between female and male callers. The least educated group were disproportionately older than the other educational levels. However, there was a striking difference in prior use of the system. With all callers, education made a big difference in reports of prior use of the service, however, for blacks, education made no difference. Regardless of educational attainment, only two percent of black callers had ever used the system before. This discovery suggests that there are factors characteristic of this ethnic group other than education which account for their low repeated useage of the system.

For blacks, education did not affect subjects inquired about but did affect cancer sites asked about. The least educated were less likely to ask about breast cancer and more likely to ask about lung cancer, probably reflecting the higher prevalence of smoking among lower educated blacks. The least educated blacks also reported more often that they first heard of the CIS through a relative (8.2%) than the most educated black callers (2.2%).

The most unexpected finding about the CIS's response to black callers was the absence of an education effect for referrals to specialized cancer centers. Education did not affect the referral of black callers as it did for the total group of callers. About 5 percent of blacks regardless of education were referred to specialized cancer centers, compared to 6.5 percent of the total least educated callers and 11.9 percent of the total most educated callers.

Hispanic Callers

The less educated Hispanic callers differed considerably from the total population of less educated callers. First, a smaller proportion of men called the CIS from the less educated group (22.6%) than from the more educated group (32.8%). Second, and surprisingly, in the least educated group, four percent of the callers said they had used the service previously but only two percent of the most educated callers reported prior usage. Therefore, the utilization gap which we identified in the total group of users was not apparent in the Hispanic callers.

Less educated Hispanics were more likely to ask about general cancer information and less likely to ask about prevention and treatment. Education did not affect the cancer site inquired about.

The less educated group were more often told to stop smoking and less frequently referred to specialized cancer centers.

Asian Callers

Overall, the Asian callers were the best educated ethnic group. Therefore, the numbers in the least educated groups were quite small. Of nearly 10,000 Asians that provided information on their ethnicitiy during the reporting period, only 99 had a grade school education, and 274 had less than a high school diploma. As with Hispanics, men in the least educated groups were even less likely to use the CIS (19.2%) than men in the most educated groups (36.6%). These less educated callers also were disproportionately older than the more educated callers. As with blacks, education did not seem to affect prior useage of the CIS.

For Asians, education affected only one subject of inquiry. Less educated Asians were less likely to ask about treatment than their more educated counterparts. Moreover, the less educated Asians were less likely to ask about cervical cancer. Conversely, they were more likely to ask about non-melanoma skin cancer. Several differences emerged between the way the less and more educated Asians first learned of the CIS. Consistent with other ethnic groups, the less educated group was more likely to use television as an information source. What was surprising, however, was that the least educated group also used newspapers more frequently than the most educated group (36.6% vs. 25.1%). The less educated group was less likely, however, to use other print sources such as brochures/pamphlets and newsletters and magazines.

There were several differences in the responses to calls from the lowest and highest educated groups of Asians. The grade school educated Asians were advised to talk to or visit a physician, to stop smoking, and to call the ACS more often than those with at least a high school diploma. On the other hand, these less educated Asians were advised to seek a second opinion, to read the literature, and to go to a specialized cancer center less often than their more educated counterparts. The calls from

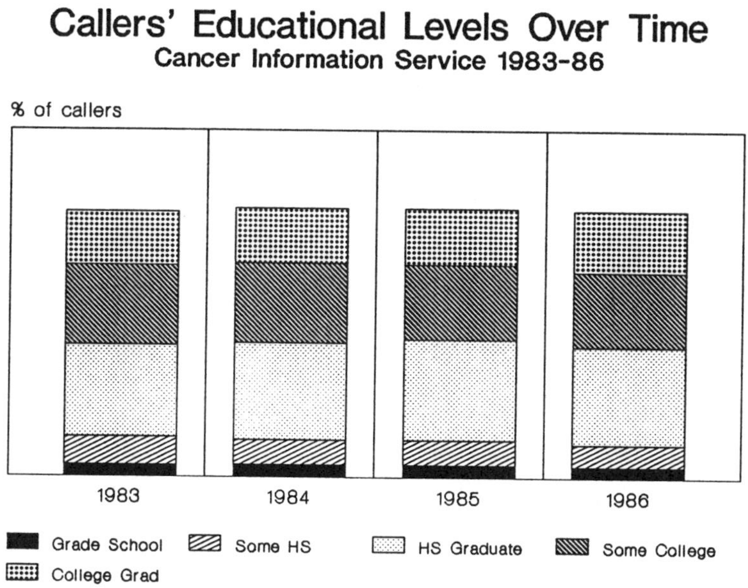

Figure 9.2

those with less education also were shorter than from those with more education.

Educational Trends

In order to examine the knowledge gap hypothesis, which suggests that the more mass media communication about a topic that flows throughout a system, the larger the gap grows, we looked for any trends in the proportion of callers from different education levels over the four years. Figure 9.2 shows that the proportions of callers in each category is reasonably stable across the four years.

The only evidence of a continuous trend is in the college graduates' small but consistent increase in proportion of calls over the four years. This evidence would suggest that sustained mediated information about the CIS has the greatest effect on the more, not the less educated groups. In general, however, these data do not support or refute the original knowledge gap hypothesis. Since the proportions of callers from the various educational strata are reasonably consistent over the four years, it is likely that awareness and utilization of the CIS depends more on motivation than on education alone or the interaction between media publicity and education. When the public want or need cancer information, they begin to perceive cancer publicity selectively, become aware of the CIS, and use the system. It may be that the more educated people have greater information resources and skills and therefore channel their motivation more effectively into use of the system.

Summary

In this chapter we focused on the information poor who are notoriously less knowledgeable about most health issues and who underutilize many of the available services, including the CIS. The dilemma for health communicators is that this group frequently is a priority target audience because it has higher incidence and mortality from many chronic diseases, including cancer. These information poor often have inadequate processing skills, are locked in an information ghetto, are fatalistic, and overdependent on television as a communication channel.

The information poor also are less healthy. They are less inclined to take preventive measures, they delay longer in seeking medical care, and they are likely to get medical care from clinics, emergency rooms, or marginal practitioners found in their neighborhoods. Consequently their survival rates for many diseases are below those for more affluent Americans.

The knowledge gap hypothesis predicts that as mass media information is infused into a social system, members with more education acquire knowledge faster than do those with relatively less education. When the knowledge gap hypothesis is applied to health topics, only part of the hypothesis appears to be supported. Gaps in health knowledge do appear between low and high SES groups at one point in time. However, increasing mass media information disseminated about that topic may actually reduce, instead of increase, the gaps.

The knowledge gap hypothesis has been attributed to characteristics of the audience, the message, and the social system. The audience of information "have nots" can be described as having inferior communication skills, an inadequate foundation of knowledge on which to expand, and fewer social network links. Message characteristics are usually discussed as some sort of ceiling or upper limit on the information which allows the information "have nots" to catch up. Social system causal factors shift the responsibility for the gaps from the individual to the social system. Design and accessibility of the system are factors accounting for its use or nonuse.

In the final section of this chapter, we analyzed the CIS database for trends in the proportion of callers from different education levels over the four years. In general, these data did not support the original knowledge gap hypothesis. We concluded that the awareness and utilization of a comprehensive communications system like the CIS depended more on motivation than on education alone or on the interaction between media publicity and education.

10

Conclusions

Naisbitt (1984) warned that we run the risk of "drowning in information but starving for knowledge." (p. 17). As early as 1970 Toffler articulated the need for new systems to allow us efficiently to store and access the enormous volume of available information. The NCI estimate that we could have a 50 percent reduction in cancer deaths by the year 2000 with better application of existing knowledge and technology (NCI, 1986a) offers powerful motivation for meeting this challenge. In this book we have examined one response to this information explosion, a comprehensive cancer communication system, the CIS. It is one of the rapidly growing number of telephone-based information/referral services which use an "800" number.

In the last twenty years, these "800" numbers, enabling toll-free, long-distance telephone calls, have unleashed a revolution in telecommunications, marketing, information services, and personal dialing habits (Yarrow, 1987). Over 400,000 of these numbers are in operation, offering such services as health information, travel reservations, financial reports, consumer goods, and emotional support. In 1986 four billion toll-free calls were answered.

Buying and selling account for the biggest use of "800" numbers. Eighty percent of the Spiegel catalogue's $820 million in sales in 1986 resulted from 14.7 million calls to its toll-free line. Holiday Inn received 19 million calls, accounting for $1 billion in hotel reservations, and Hertz-Rent-A-Car received 16 million calls in 1986 (Yarrow, 1987).

Toll-free numbers are also used to improve public relations. Large corporations such as IBM and DuPont have product-information numbers. Many government and nonprofit agencies, other than NCI, use "800" numbers to provide a wide range of information. For example, in 1986, the Internal Revenue Service took 40 million toll-free calls from taxpayers.

Emotional support is another well-known "800" service. Hotlines offer support and advice to drug abusers, parents of missing children and many others. For example, volunteers provide around-the-clock crisis intervention on the Chicago-based National Adolescent Suicide Hotline and the National Runaway Switchboard.

These telephone information services are one of the responses to the challenge of designing systems to efficiently store and disseminate information to the public. The CIS is one of the most comprehensive and mature of these services, having started in 1976. Consequently this analysis of its development, operations, and evaluation offers valuable insights to anyone facing the prospect of taming the information tide for the public. For this final chapter, we take the perspective of the communicator who is charged with disseminating information and offer those insights we gained from reviewing the literature on the public's search for health information and analyzing the extensive data from the CIS.

Traditional Information Dissemination Approaches

Traditionally communicators have used a variety of channels to disseminate health information. Some of the more common approaches have included public service announcements (PSAs) on television and radio, print advertisements, posters, pamphlets, and brochures. These approaches are characterized by a centralized source pre-packaging information and sending it in a linear manner to a set of passive receivers. Communicators learned over time that these approaches were not very effective unless the needs of the audience and their reactions to the materials were considered. Hence, needs assessment research and pretesting of materials became commonplace. Still, in many cases, the results were disappointing. Many evaluation studies showed that few of the target audience could recall the messages or their main ideas and many misconceptions persisted. Most importantly, the desired behavior change often did not take place. As a result, many of the early communicators decried the ignorance and apathy of the public.

Dervin interpreted these disappointing outcomes differently. She argued that people are quite active information seekers if they believe they need the information. Pre-packaged information often fails to answer the critical questions they have. In fact, she suggested that people create their own information, and only seek more when they experience gaps in their understanding. There is considerable evidence of these "constructions" or idiosyncratic interpretations, especially of illnesses and their etiology.

Even when people are able to recall the official message about a health issue (e.g., high blood pressure has no symptoms), they often fail to apply it to themselves, preferring their own personal interpretations.

Unique Capabilities of the CIS

A comprehensive communication system such as the CIS is uniquely capable of meeting these individualized needs for information. It is one of the few information sources that does not predetermine what information to disseminate, but allows the user to define his/her own information needs. Indeed, the data from the system demonstrate the enormous diversity of these needs. Over 56 different codes are used to describe the nature of the inquiries, and there is considerable variety within each code. Another advantage of this type of system is that it acts as a gatekeeper to control both the volume and quality of information and, most importantly for a health topic, translate the information into a comprehensible form for the lay person.

A comprehensive communication system such as the CIS incorporates important communication principles. For example, it is well known that mass media are most effective in stimulating awareness of an issue while interpersonal communication is much more effective in persuading someone to change attitudes and/or behavior. The CIS relies on mass media, often television PSAs, to stimulate an information search or to alert a searcher to the existence of the service. The telephone provides the technology to link the caller and the information specialist in an interpersonal encounter where the interaction is both personalized and anonymous. Moreover, the information dissemination which occurs is not a linear process with a centralized source sending pre-determined information to a passive receiver. Instead the interpersonal communication is quite interactive and dynamic. For example, users often call repeatedly as they move through stages of the disease and their information needs change. The entire system also is interactive in the sense that it both directs information seeking to specific issues and reacts to pressures for information from its users, as illustrated by the interleukin-2 example in Chapter Eight.

The telephone is a critical element in such a comprehensive communications system. It enables a personalized service to be delivered to the masses. Unlike most communication technologies, the telephone is low-cost, almost universally available, and simple to use. At the same time, such technological innovations as an "800" number, expanded WATS, and advanced WATS service have been added to this system without burdening the individual user. The system does use other media as well. Television, radio, newspapers, magazines, posters, brochures, and pamphlets are used to publicize the service. Often written information materials are sent as follow-up to callers to reinforce the telephone information and to provide a source that can be referred to repeatedly. This type of printed material, unlike the unsolicited pamphlet or brochure, does not have to compete with many other attractive messages for the person's attention. Because it has been requested in an interpersonal interaction and supported by encouragement to read it, it enjoys a high probability of being read.

Insights from Analyses of Different User Groups

An examination of the process individuals use when trying to acquire health information may help the communicator design a system to optimally meet the needs of its users. Although this book has focused on cancer, our model of the health information acquisition process should apply to other topics as well. Not all users search for health information in the same way. As people move along the disease continuum from primary prevention through symptoms and diagnosis to treatment and rehabilitation or continuing care their information needs change. In the analysis of the CIS data, the position along this disease continuum seemed to be a better predictor of the type of information search than did any of the demographic classifications available. Members of the general public who did not have any immediate personal involvement with cancer appeared to need an external stimulus like a television message about prevention, smoking, or other risk factors to initiate a limited information search. Most of their calls were simple requests to order publications they had seen advertised on television. For many of these general public callers, the information search probably ended when the booklet sent to them was read. Yet reaching this group with accurate information is critical because the beliefs and attitudes they form at this stage of involvement with the disease will influence the way they might perceive their own symptoms and seek and respond to treatment should they progress along this disease continuum in the future. For these callers, it is likely that the benefits of seeking the information outweighed the "costs." The materials were free, the telephone call was free, and one's anonymity could be protected. Since there was little involvement with the disease at this point, the anxiety should not have been high. It is also likely that no other information sources were consulted.

People with symptoms, however, approach the information acquisition process quite differently. The stimulus is probably their actual physical symptoms accompanied by a labeling of these symptoms as potentially cancer-related. Hence, the stimulus is a much more powerful one, creating greater uncertainty coupled with more anxiety. This information search is likely to be much more prolonged and complex than the general public's search. However, for some people, perhaps up to one third of the population, the search may be truncated quickly at the cost/benefit comparison. If the perceived "costs" include financial, social, and emotional distress, the symptomatic person may deny the problem or delay the search indefinitely. For some of these people, the denial or delay may be interrupted later by strong media messages which stimulate the information search to begin once again. These information seekers are likely to use many sources, probably beginning with informal contacts through their own social networks. There is some evidence that the density of those networks may affect their utilization of other sources, such as an information/referral service. Those people who have a very dense network are less likely to use external sources, either because they do not know they exist, or because they do not perceive that they need further help. On the other hand, these informal sources often encourage symptomatic people to seek medical care.

Cancer patients and their family/friends, however, have undoubtedly been recycling through the information acquisition process throughout their progression along the disease continuum. Of all groups studied, they have the most intense need for information. Many studies have shown that information seeking, particularly immediately following diagnosis, relieves anxiety and restores a sense of control to the patient or their family member. Although the physician is generally the primary source of information for patients, there is ample evidence of the difficulties both patients and their families experience in getting answers to their questions from the physician alone. Physicians may be unavailable to answer questions or incapable of or unwilling to give explanations that patients and their families can understand. Therefore, we think that the most active information seeking occurs for these people who often report learning of the CIS through the white pages in the telephone book or other sources which require an active search and who use the CIS repeatedly more often than any other group of users.

An examination of the way in which a comprehensive communications system such as the CIS responds to its users also offers insights to the communication specialist. Behavioral suggestions are usually given to callers. From the user surveys we examined, there is strong evidence that the suggestions requiring little cost, either financial or emotional, are generally followed, again showing the power of the interpersonal interaction in stimulating behavioral actions. Those suggestions which required the caller to follow-up on a referral, either to a physician or other resource, were ignored more often. However, even physician referrals, if made to callers with symptoms, were generally followed. Moreover, those callers who reported that their most important question was answered in their call to the CIS were the most likely to comply with the behavioral suggestion. All of these results reinforce Dervin's concept of active information seekers who try to fill gaps in their own understanding and who appear more likely to follow behavioral suggestions when their understanding is more complete.

Insights from Analyses of the Demographic Characteristics of Callers

Even though stage of involvement with the disease was the best predictor of information seeking, certain trends did emerge from the demographic analyses which should be useful in helping others reach target audiences. Many more women used this information system than did men. This skewed distribution may only apply to health issues since women traditionally play the role of information gatherers for the family's health. No data on gender distributions for non-health related information services could be found with which to compare our data. For some of the more critical information needs, such as treatment, the proportion of male callers increased.

The age distribution of the callers appeared to reinforce the influence of saliency in determining who uses this information service. Middle-aged persons (40 to 60 years old) called at higher rates than their representation in the population would predict. Since cancer incidence increases with age, it is likely that the saliency of the issue also increases with age, motivating more calls in the older age groups. This trend did not hold, though, for those aged 60 and over, who call in the same proportion as their population figures would predict. What we think is happening for these ages is that information seeking often is handled by adult children rather than by the elderly themselves. The data for cancer patients and their family/friends strongly support this explanation. All of these findings suggest that communicators also may need to target their messages at support networks surrounding the targeted individual.

As expected from previous research, education is the variable which most strongly determines use of this information/referral system. The dilemma for communicators is clear. Those least likely to get information through other traditional communication channels are also less likely to use information/referral systems such as the CIS. Unfortunately the data do not help us understand whether these less educated people are unaware of the service, or are aware but choose not to use it. This relationship between low education and low utilization remained unchanged during the four years of CIS data examined in this book. Thus, the knowledge gap hypothesis was not supported, i.e., the publicity surrounding the CIS over time has not increased these knowledge and utilization gaps. Yet these gaps have not narrowed in spite of four years of promotion efforts. Certainly this underutilization problem is a serious one that needs to be addressed by anyone involved in an information-referral service. The promotion of the system must address the value the potential user assigns to information and stimulate motivation for engaging in an information search. Similar to the impact of education, ethnicity influences the utilization of the service. Asians and whites use the system disproportionately more frequently than blacks, Hispanics, and American Indians. Even within ethnic groups, however, education continues to affect utilization. For each ethnic group examined, the less educated members used the system less frequently than the more educated members. For only one of these ethnic groups, blacks, are there any data to suggest what level of awareness of the service exists. Blacks reported greater awareness of the CIS than whites but less utilization. If an information service is to be truly representative, communicators must find ways of reaching and motivating these underusers. The dilemma, however, is whether the education or the ethnicity is the more important characteristic to consider when targeting to these audiences.

Insights from Analyses of Promotion Efforts

Providing the information service is not enough. It must also be promoted. We have demonstrated in our analysis how important an understanding of user groups is to these promotions. Planned promotions should target specific users, based on stage along the disease continuum, demographic, or psychographic characteristics, so that messages can be specific, motivating, and sent through appropriate channels. General, diffuse messages are unlikely to be very effective. We have demonstrated the effectiveness of such techniques as including an action step in messages (e.g., call 1-800-4-CANCER for additional information), using highly credible sources, and targeting to specific sub-groups of the population. One conclusion that is strongly supported by these data is the ability of mass media to stimulate use of an information/referral system. In all of the campaigns illustrated using the CIS telephone number, there has been a dramatic increase in resulting calls. Even more dramatic has been the response to media coverage of unplanned events involving cancer. Whether a famous person's experience with cancer or publicity surrounding a new treatment or cause of cancer, these events seem to set an agenda for the public to seek more information on the topic. In the past ten years, the CIS has matured from a fledgling, passive information system struggling to cope with demands for a proper national evaluation to a confident, active information service working hard to stimulate as well as respond to the public's information needs.

Development of Foreign Cancer Information Services

Over the years, the United States was not the only country to recognize consumers' needs for cancer information. Several other countries have developed communications systems similar to the CIS. Some were modeled after the U.S. system, and others developed completely unaware of the CIS's existence.

In England, the British Association of Cancer United Patients (BACUP) was launched in October, 1985. BACUP was formed as a three-way partnership between patients living with cancer, their families, and the health professionals who look after them. BACUP's information service is operated by five specially trained senior nurses, all experienced in cancer care. Over 15,000 inquiries were handled by BACUP in its first year. BACUP has developed a three-part evaluation system: (1) a telephone monitoring system—a call-logging device which provides information on the number and duration of calls; (2) recording inquiry information including sex and age of callers, location, nature of the inquiries, and the information provided; and (3) a user survey sent to callers to measure their satisfaction with the service. The BACUP program was modeled after the CIS and BACUP staff visited regional CIS offices while planning their program. They also invited the CIS project director at NCI to spend a week in their offices to provide technical assistance prior to full-scale program implementation.

In France, the cancer telephone service has a different mission. Ecoute Cancer, begun in 1982, is a non-directive listening service which maintains both parties' anonymity. This service does not provide medical information. The objective is to let callers express themselves and confide problems. Social workers and one lawyer staff the telephones. Each caller is given a unique number and a call record form is completed, so if users call repeatedly, they do not have to repeat their history. The service has collected over 20,000 records. Up to 40 percent of all calls are classified as "silent calls," meaning that the person on the other end does not talk at all. The staff is instructed to stay on the line with these callers offering such supportive comments as, "I know this must be difficult for you to talk about."

The Belgian program, Hallo Kanker, began in 1984 and has received over 4,000 calls. A "social nurse" and an oncologist are on the staff. The goals of the system are to provide accurate, comprehensible cancer information and psychological assistance for callers. Germany's program, KID, was also modeled after the CIS in the U.S. It began as a small, pilot program in October, 1985, and was fully staffed with ten full-time employees and 20 part-time volunteers by July, 1986. It has received over 15,000 calls. Germany also has a private cancer association in Bonn, Deutsche Krebshiffer, established in 1974. This organization recently started a computer-based information service which received 12,000 telephone inquiries, 1,320 letters, and 480 personal contacts in 1986.

Other countries, including the Netherlands, operate similar systems, and Israel plans to open a cancer information service in the near future.

All of the existing services collect some data on their calls. In the following section, we will compare and contrast these data to the data from the CIS. Figure 10.1 compares the proportion of calls coming from different types of users of these cancer information services. Clearly, the U.S. system serves considerably different users than the other systems. More calls are placed to the CIS from the general public. In the other countries, however, the program primarily serves cancer patients and their family/friends. This difference is probably influenced by the mass media promotion of the CIS, especially the offers of prevention-oriented materials available by calling the CIS.

In all the countries where data have been collected on the programs, women callers outnumber men. In the U.S. and Belgium, women outnumber men three to one, but in Germany the proportions are closer to two to one.

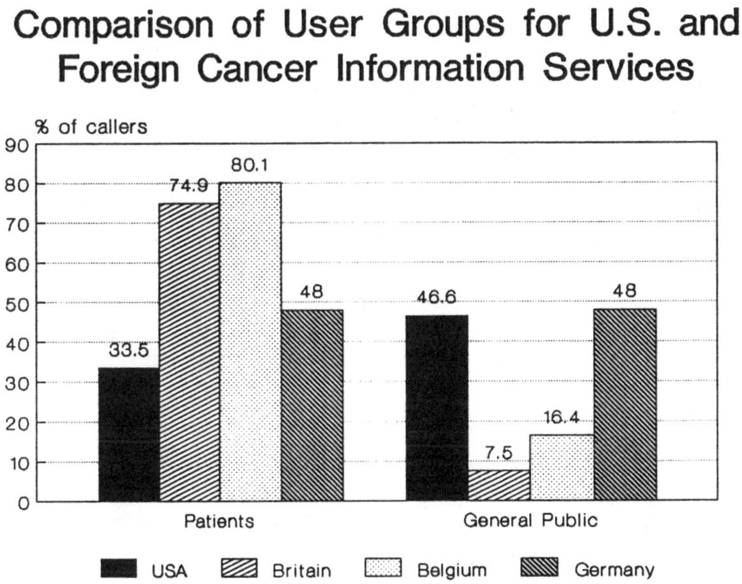

Figure 10.1

The breast was the cancer site most frequently asked about by callers to all the systems who had collected information on sites. Intestinal or colon/rectum was the cancer site inquired about next most often.

Future Directions for the Cancer Information Service

The CIS continues to grow and to examine its potential role in the primary prevention and treatment of cancer. In 1987, five grants were awarded by NCI for research on cancer communications. Two of the grantees responded to knowledge and utilization gaps by studying ways to reach underserved populations with cancer information. The University of Maryland project is examining use of the CIS by black Americans to explore communications issues relative to the non-use of the CIS by this group, and to recommend strategies for health communicators in order to narrow the knowledge gap in this population. The Illinois Cancer Council in Chicago is studying the information needs, patterns of information seeking behavior, and use of cancer-related information among cancer patient users of the CIS, and comparing these data with data from a control group of cancer patients.

Roswell Park Memorial Institute in Buffalo, New York, is studying the effectiveness of targeted communications compared to non-targeted communications that encourage quitting smoking. In their first study, they are testing the effectiveness of a radio/television campaign targeted to young female smokers with young children in motivating them to want to quit smoking and to call the CIS to obtain help in quitting. The second study involves random assignment to subjects who call the CIS regarding quitting smoking of one of three quit smoking manuals, one that is specifically designed for mothers of children under six, as compared to two "standard" manuals. The quitting behavior of these callers will be measured six months following their call to the CIS.

The remaining two research projects explore an expanded and more aggressive role for the CIS. The University of California at Los Angeles is transforming the CIS to a more active system which targets particular subgroups of callers for specific cancer control messages irrespective of their initial reason for calling the CIS. Moreover, they are using the CIS to reinforce recommended behaviors through follow-up telephone calls. Specifically, they are conducting a randomized field experiment involving over 3,000 female callers for the purpose of evaluating the CIS as a mechanism for promoting the use of mammography for breast cancer screening. The following three groups are included in their study: (1) standard practice group in which information and recommendations about mammography are disseminated upon request; (2) active promotion of mammography to all eligible female callers 50 years or older, irrespective of the caller's initial reason for calling the CIS; and (3) the same active promotion as in group two plus a two-week reinforcement interview to encourage adherence to the mammography guidelines. The effectiveness of these interventions will be measured at six months with self-reported utilization data and audits of billing records at participating mammography facilities for a subset of callers.

The Fred Hutchinson Cancer Research Center in Seattle, Washington, is also studying an innovative application for the CIS. They are determining the effectiveness of a hotline intervention for smoking cessation with blue collar smokers who are likely to be heavy smokers and difficult to reach. They are enrolling these smokers through three worksites in the Seattle, Washington area by promotion of a CIS hotline that will provide smoking cessation messages. A special smoking cessation hotline, added to the existing CIS service, was designed for the target population in order to help telephone staff identify a caller's stage in the cessation process and to provide appropriate information, coping strategies, and materials. Evaluation for this project will consist of interview data at the first call, one month later, and at six and twelve month intervals. The twelve month follow-up will be supplemented with biochemical validation. Appendix F lists complete addresses for the communications research grantees described above.

The results of these research projects may signal a new phase in the development of the CIS with the service assuming an expanded, more aggressive role in health promotion.

Appendix A

The History and Development of the CIS

Program Origins

Cancer has been recognized as a major health problem in the United States for many years. In 1928 legislation was introduced in the United States Senate to authorize the National Academy of Sciences to:

> investigate the means and methods for affording Federal aid in discovering a cure for cancer.

Nine years later the National Cancer Institute (NCI) was created by Congress. However, substantial Federal interest in cancer really became evident in 1970 when Senator Ralph Yarborough (D-Texas) introduced legislation to establish a "National Cancer Authority" to head up a national effort to eliminate cancer. One month later, in the 1971 State of the Union Message, President Richard Nixon called for an additional appropriation of $100 million to control cancer. On December 23, 1971, the President signed the National Cancer Act (PL 92–218) initiating the National Cancer Program under the leadership of the NCI. Since then the annual appropration for the NCI has steadily increased until today when the budget (excluding AIDS) exceeds $1.1 billion. With this unprecedented growth in Federal support for cancer research, the problem of how to transfer existing and anticipated new knowledge into effective cancer prevention and control behavior by the public and health professionals began to receive attention.

The NCI has had a major focus on cancer communications for many years. Within the Institute there are two major sources of support for such programming: the Office of Cancer Communications (OCC), part of the

NCI Director's office, and what is currently called the Division of Cancer Prevention and Control (DCPC), formerly the Division of Cancer Control and Rehabilitation (DCCR). The Cancer Information Service (CIS) was conceived by OCC and developed jointly by DCCR and OCC. Throughout its history the CIS has received funding support and program leadership from DCPC, while OCC staff have provided program leadership, support and resources, technical guidance, and integration with other Institute communications efforts.

The basic concept of the CIS program is a network of regional offices which solicit and respond to inquiries on any aspect of cancer from users including the general public, symptomatic individuals, cancer patients and their families and friends, and health professionals. The regional offices form a national "network" under NCI's direction which not only meets the immediate needs of those calling each office, but also serves as a conduit for providing in a rapid and effective manner new information derived from NCI research. The principal means for receiving inquiries has been the use of toll-free telephone lines. CIS offices are open a minimum of eight hours per day including the core hours of 9:00 A.M. to 4:00 P.M. local time, Monday through Friday. After business hours, weekends and holidays, callers are greeted by a tape message referring the caller back to the CIS during regular business hours or to a national office which provides some after-hours and weekend coverage. Regional offices generally serve the population of the state in which they are located, although some have expanded to serve surrounding states as well. A national CIS, under the direction of OCC staff, provides coverage to all parts of the country not served by a regional CIS and back-up coverage for regional offices.

The regional Cancer Information Service offices have been funded throughout their history largely under contract with the Federal government. The original solicitation for proposals to begin CIS programs was issued on September 23, 1974, and noted that:

> The Strategic Plan of the National Cancer Program states that research advances as well as existing knowledge must be translated into effective action through communication to the public and to health professionals. This is intended to reduce the incidence, morbidity, and mortality from cancer.

Therein lies the basic goal statement of the CIS: to contribute to a reduction in cancer rates through an effective program of communications to the public and health professionals. That goal statement has basically remained intact throughout the history of the CIS. However, as the program has evolved over time, a decided emphasis on communications programs for the public, rather than health professionals, has become apparent.

At the time the program began, the NCI was in the process of recognizing "comprehensive cancer centers" under the authority of the National Cancer Act. These centers were to be places of excellence in clinical and basic research, education and training, and patient care. They were also expected by NCI to play a significant cancer control role within their communities through demonstration and outreach programs, including the dissemination of information to professional and lay audiences. Because of this mandate, NCI decided to actively support the development of information and education programs in these centers. Thus, the original request for proposals was for a limited competition directed only at the 17 comprehensive cancer centers designated at the time and with the intention that multiple contracts would be awarded.

It should be pointed out that this entire program was established in a traditionally basic science organization (the National Institutes of Health (NIH)) to be carried out by basic and clinical research organizations (comprehensive cancer centers). Its concept was controversial and was greeted skeptically at first on all fronts. It had to be "sold" first to cancer center directors at meetings in late 1973 and early 1974 and then to the NIH Director and his immediate staff.

As it turned out, one of the CIS program's greatest strengths derived from its beginnings at NCI and the comprehensive cancer centers- the most credible, pre-eminent cancer research organizations in the world. Their credibility strengthened the CIS program, even though sometimes it was an unwelcome stepchild at its own institution. The NCI and cancer centers also gave the CIS staff access to the best and most up-to-date cancer information at a time when research progress was changing cancer care at a dazzling pace.

Elements of the CIS Program

Documentation related to funding the original contracts tends to describe the objectives of the program in terms of establishing the mechanisms necessary to have an effective communications program, rather than to delineate specific expectations as a result of establishing these mechanisms. Thus, the only objective stated in the initial contract statement of work for all CIS programs notes:

> a communications office is being established as a focal point to which the layman and his physician can turn for information, help and advice. Information/education office staff shall develop materials and resources required to conduct program activities

In general, the programmatic elements of the CIS can be divided into three general parts: resources, services, and evaluation, the various components of which are discussed more fully in this Appendix. "Resources" includes the development of information and education materials, as well as the development of subject matter files and directories of agencies and organizations that provide services to cancer patients and their families. Service refers to the actual activity associated with providing information to CIS users, including mechanisms and processes for response to inquiries and ancillary support needs such as promotion, policy development, and staff training. Evaluation is self-explanatory, and its various components and results are covered in detail throughout this book.

Early Program Expectations

At this point, a discussion of some of the early program expectations that subsequently shaped the nature of the CIS is appropriate:

1. It is quite clear from the original work statement outlined by NCI that the CIS was intended to meet the multiple cancer information needs of the population. With that was an implied expectation that the program would result in measurable changes in overall public knowledge, attitudes, and practices related to cancer. This implied expectation subsequently resulted in a measure of stress for program managers at the national and regional office as attempts were made in the early days to "prove" the success of the program and to justify its continuation. It was not until later in the program that the ability to measure such changes in a way to permit linkage with CIS as the change agent was acknowledged as unrealistic and more attainable evaluation goals were specified.

2. A letter dated July 17, 1975 from Dr. Frank Rauscher, then Director of NCI, to each of the comprehensive cancer center directors noted that the CIS would be a highly visible activity due to its nature as a public service and its use of the mass media for promotional purposes. With this letter Dr. Rauscher clearly indicated high expectations for the CIS. But

he also indirectly raised the specter that its very visibility might also make it a source of potential public embarrassment to the institutions housing each office. Accordingly, each of the CIS offices underwent a period during which it developed operating policies and procedures to assure high quality services and to avoid such embarrassment. The resulting policies in some offices (e.g., physician referral) were more restrictive than in others depending on the degree of concern generated in each institution about this new source of visibility.

3. Dr. Rauscher's letter also conveyed another message which had major implications for the long-term future of CIS. He set forth the idea that while the CIS was being created to assist each center's informational/educational efforts,

> we all must constantly guard not only against use of the individual offices and the entire network for public relations purposes, but against even the appearance of such use.

It is true that the centers' public relations programs have serendipitously benefited from the CIS. But this lack of ability to utilize the CIS for direct public relations or fund raising purposes may also have diminished the interest of some cancer center directors in firmly establishing the CIS office as an integral part of their institution. Whether true or not, this policy was a far-sighted one which was cited often when demonstrating to community agencies that the CIS was truly a public service, and not a ploy to serve the public relations and patient recruitment interests of the centers.

4. It is also clear from Dr. Rauscher's letter and the initial statement of work for the CIS that the intent from the outset of the CIS program was to have a true "network." However, there also was a heavy emphasis on fulfilling center's obligations to provide information/education programs within their own service areas. To a much lesser extent, references were made to participating in an overall national communications effort and contributing to the overall cancer control mission of the NCI. The assumption may have been that establishing a number of regional offices would automatically result in meeting the entire nation's cancer information needs without having to specify any other means for directly achieving this result. Thus, few mechanisms for ongoing interaction and communications between regional CIS offices were stipulated in the original contracts. Fortunately, funds were provided for periodic national meetings and some of the more far-sighted leaders in the early days es-

tablished other mechanisms and operating procedures to encourage national interaction.

5. Finally, it was intended that the initial CIS offices would eventually provide coverage for all geographic areas within the continental United States. Initially, it was thought that each CIS would cover its own state and then expand into contiguous states. This expectation left room for wide variation in expansion capabilities of individual CIS offices. For example, the Connecticut CIS had virtually no room for expansion of any sort, except to Rhode Island, because the other states surrounding it already had regional CIS offices. The Massachusetts CIS, on the other hand, eventually expanded to cover Maine, New Hampshire, and Vermont. In the West and Southwest, expansion was certainly possible, but not often feasible. It was suggested, for example, that the Texas CIS expand to cover all of New Mexico, Oklahoma, Arkansas, and Louisiana. But the magnitude of the effort involved in covering Texas and its 254 counties alone exhausted the fiscal and personnel resources of the Texas contract. Thus, it became apparent that it was an unrealistic expectation at that time that all of the country would be serviced by a regional CIS office.

Program Implementation

Developmental activities in the regional offices began in the spring and summer of 1975, following the award of the first contracts to the 17 then-designated comprehensive cancer centers. Originally, it was believed that most of the CIS offices would begin providing services in January of 1976. This prediction proved to be highly optimistic, as can be seen by the early program data presented in the accompanying table. The table shows the number of offices reporting user volume information to NCI through September, 1976. Only those offices showing more than 25 calls per month were considered operational. Moreover, on the advice of NCI (and many others) most CIS offices utilized some type of phase-in approach in which publicity efforts were staggered to allow the service to obtain experience from a limited geographic base before expanding coverage to the entire service area. Thus, full access to a CIS by the majority of the population being served probably did not begin to occur until late 1976 or early 1977.

In 1978 the contracts were renewed for an additional three years for each of the incumbents and two newly designated comprehensive centers

Offices Reporting User Volume Information to NCI
January–September, 1976

Month in 1976	Number of offices operational
January	0
February	1
March	1
April	2
May	3
June	5
July	9
August	12
September	13

were given first-time contracts. About that time an investigator-initiated grant application also received an award for a CIS-type program and was eventually included in the network. In 1982, 17 contracts were awarded following an open competition. Fourteen incumbents received new awards, while four did not receive further NCI funding. Two new awards were made to cancer centers which had operated CIS-type programs in the past. One new award was made to a cancer center which had never operated this type of program before. A fourth competition for Federal contracts in 1985 and some private funding has resulted in the current configuration of the CIS in 1988 with 25 regional offices.

It is important to appreciate that despite a basically generic contract for all CIS regional offices, major differences have existed between individual offices in terms of both resources and program capability. For example, offices which served larger population bases (e.g., Florida and Georgia, covered by an office located at the University of Miami) tended to have larger budgets for staff, travel, promotion, etc., than did those serving smaller states. As was seen in the data presented throughout this book, the CIS has gone from these modest beginnings to a highly successful, well established program of the National Cancer Institute. The program was reviewed in 1987 and approved for a fifth recompetition which will extend its lifetime an additional five years, thus making it a very longstanding Federal commitment when compared to most government programs.

Program Evaluation

The preliminary work undertaken in the years between the inception of the CIS network in 1975 and the implementation of the national evaluation in 1983 heavily influenced the nature of the resulting evaluation which is reported in this book.

In this section, we describe the role that evaluation plays in the program, its evolution to the point that a standardized evaluation was put in place, and the general content of the overall evaluation plan.

The importance of evaluation for any program of this type, scope and cost cannot be overstated. Evaluation can and should be used as a means of determining whether program goals and objectives are being accomplished, and as a management tool throughout the program's lifespan to continually assess and improve the operational aspects of service delivery.

Early Evaluation Efforts

The NCI recognized the need for this important element of the program from the outset. The first official references to evaluation appeared in the performance specifications issued by NCI for the first CIS contracts in 1974:

> Evaluation shall be incorporated as part of the office activities to determine, both qualitatively and quantitatively, the impact of the office on the center's constituency. Evaluation efforts shall be designed to provide the information which a center requires to improve and modify its communications program and which is required to identify successful programs which might be transferred to other centers

The workscope went on to state that institutions wishing to operate CIS offices must have the capability to determine the demographic characteristics of the population being served by the CIS and be able to compare these with the population as a whole. The population of each service area also had to be compared to "high risk" profiles for cancer. Media through which the population learned of the program were to be determined, as was user satisfaction with the program and the information provided, and action taken by users based on its recommendations. The specifications also noted that, if feasible, data on changes in cancer screening, staging and referral patterns should be incorporated into the program, although it was made clear that there were no funds available for "detailed referral and biometric studies."

While the intellectual commitment to evaluation by both the government and CIS network staff was present from the outset, it quickly became evident that two major issues would impact negatively on the development of an evaluation for the program. First, the vast majority of all NCI contract funds were allocated for the purpose of providing information services and developing the resources needed to do so effectively. Many CIS regional offices had no funds for evaluation in their contracts, and for those few that did it was minimal. Second, there was no contractual requirement and, at the outset, little impetus for developing a standardized, national evaluation that would allow for common data collection and comparison among all CIS offices.

Development of a National Program Evaluation

NCI staff realized early in the program's development that a number of CIS regional offices desired a national evaluation program and thus made efforts to establish an evaluation with input from all CIS offices. In November 1975, an Evaluation Task Force (ETF) was established consisting of NCI staff, several CIS regional office evaluation and program staff, and outside consultants. The ETF was charged with developing a national evaluation plan, beginning with defining a common data set for documenting inquiries to the system (which, as noted earlier, were expected to begin in early 1976). The Task Force reported its initial plans during a national CIS meeting in March, 1976. While there was some agreement on many aspects of the proposed system, there was also disagreement, particularly on those aspects related to obtaining information on user demographics and/or other user characteristics. Since there was no contractual obligation to participate in a national evaluation system and because NCI chose not to articulate a policy to that effect, the net result of this first ETF plan was that those centers wishing to use the documentation system did so (often modifying it according to their own interests) and the others did not.

This was to be the first of several unsuccessful attempts between 1976 and 1982 to put a national evaluation plan into place. During that period a number of simple reporting systems were devised and put into place, although there were no real quality control checks, documentation, or training programs to accompany them. As a result, the early years of program evaluation were characterized by each office doing largely what it wished (or not) with a few pieces of "standardized" data being kept by most offices and reported to NCI. No truly reliable national data existed to describe the overall program except, perhaps, the total number of inquiries and their type (i.e., telephone, mail, or walk-in).

In 1982, two things happened that finally resulted in the implementation of a national CIS program evaluation. First, a later version of the original ETF completed its work on designing a standardized system that incorporated much of the previous ETF's work, while adding some important and creative new features. Second, the recently renewed NCI contracts for the CIS offices contained a mandatory requirement for participation in a national evaluation and NCI backed up this requirement with the funds necessary to see that the system was properly implemented.

Ironically, the evaluation system that was eventually put in place was largely made up of the same basic elements defined in the original statement-of-work and early ETF plans. Obviously, many things had been learned in the intervening years, especially about such things as wording questions, what data were important for management purposes, and the need for assuring data consistency across CIS offices, to name a few.

In general, a three-part evaluation was put in place: a common inquiry documentation system (called the Call Record Form); a user survey; and a quality control program. The first two are the sources of the majority of the data presented in this book. The quality control program addressed the critical importance of the information being presented by CIS staff in response to an inquiry and was discussed in detail in Chapter 2.

The success of the CIS program has depended to a large extent on the results of this national evaluation; its very existence today is a direct result. In the late 1970s and the early 1980s, the CIS program was heavily criticized because it was thought to be expensive and to have little data to demonstrate its accomplishments. When approval was reluctantly given by NCI's scientific advisors in 1982 to extend the program an additional three years until 1985, it was made very clear that solid measures of its accomplishments would be a prerequisite for any further extensions of program funding. When the initial evaluation data were presented in 1984, the same group of scientific advisors (many of whom were critical in the past) gave the program their enthusiastic support. Indeed, these evaluation data have been instrumental in obtaining future funding approvals for CIS through 1994, at which time the program will be twenty years old.

In the more immediate sense, the evaluation has proved invaluable at both the national and local levels for program management purposes.

It has enabled offices to track call volume in ways that allow for more rational staffing patterns to evolve; to track public response to specific promotion or media events that generate calls; to monitor the effects of changes in technology (e.g. "expanded 800" service, discussed in Chapter 2) on call volume; to compare data among offices that provide a basis for technical advice and consultation; and, finally, to share the CIS "experience" with others in a more objective and useful manner.

Appendix B

List of CIS Offices and Areas of Coverage, 1988

National Cancer Institute

Project Officer, Cancer Information Service
National Cancer Institute
Building 31, 10A29
9000 Rockville Pike
Bethesda, MD 20892
(301) 496-6631

Alabama

Cancer Information Service
Comprehensive Cancer Center
University of Alabama at Birmingham
1918 University Blvd., Rm. 108
University Station
Birmingham, AL 35294
(205) 934-6614

California—UCLA

Cancer Information Service
Jonsson Comprehensive Cancer Center of California
1100 Glendon Ave., Suite 711
Los Angeles, CA 90024
(213) 206-0278

California—USC

Cancer Information Service
USC Office of Cancer Communications
1721 Griffin Ave., Suite 205
Los Angeles, CA 90031
(213) 224-7371

Colorado

Cancer Information Service
Penrose Hospital
P.O. Box 7021
Colorado Springs, CO 80933
(719) 630-5271

Connecticut

Cancer Information Service
Yale Comprehensive Cancer Center
333 Cedar St., LEPH 139
P.O. Box 3333
New Haven, CT 06510
(203) 785-6347

Florida (and Georgia)

Cancer Information Service
Papanicolaou Comprehensive Cancer Center
P.O. Box 016960, D8-4
Room 4035
Miami, FL 33101
(305) 548-4820

Hawaii

Cancer Information Service
Cancer Research Center of Hawaii
1236 Lauhala St., Rm. 502
Honolulu, HI 96813
(808) 548-8775

Illinois

Cancer Information Service
Illinois Cancer Council
36 Wabash Ave., Suite 700
Chicago, IL 60603
(312) 346-9813, Ext. 328

Kentucky

Kentucky Cancer Information Service
Markey Cancer Center
800 Rose St.
Lexington, KY 40536-0093
(606) 233-6545

Maryland

Johns Hopkins Cancer Information Service
550 N. Broadway, Room 307
Baltimore, MD 21205
(301) 955-3636

Massachusetts (and Maine, New Hampshire, Vermont)

Cancer Information Service
Dana-Farber Cancer Institute
44 Binney St.
Boston, MA 02115
(617) 732-3154

Michigan

Cancer Information Service
Comprehensive Cancer Center of Metropolitan Detroit
110 East Warren Ave.
Detroit, MI 48201
(313) 833-0710, Ext. 247

Minnesota (and North and South Dakota)

Cancer Information Service
American Cancer Society
3316 West 66th Street
Minneapolis, MN 55435
(612) 925-6336

Missouri

Cancer Information Service
Boone Hospital Center
1600 E. Broadway
Columbia, MO 65201
(314) 875-3506

New York City (and Northern New Jersey)

Cancer Information Service
Memorial Sloan-Kettering Cancer Center
Office of Cancer Communications
1275 York Ave.
New York, NY 10021
(212) 207-3537

New York State

Cancer Information Service
Roswell Park Memorial Institute
666 Elm Street
Buffalo, NY 14263
(716) 845-3115

North Carolina

Duke Cancer Information Service
Duke Comprehensive Cancer Center
Erwin Square, Suite 10
2020 W. Main St.
Durham, NC 27705
(919) 286-5515

Ohio

Cancer Information Service
Ohio State Comprehensive Cancer Center
101 A Hamilton Hall
1645 Neil Ave.
Columbus, OH 43210
(614) 292-1382

Oklahoma

Oklahoma Cancer Information Service
13439 N. Broadway Extension, Suite 222
Oklahoma City, OK 73114
(405) 755-6245

Pennsylvania (and Southern New Jersey and Delaware)

Cancer Information Service
Fox Chase Cancer Center
430A Rhawn St.
Philadelphia, PA 19111
(215) 728-3110

Tennessee

Cancer Information Service of Tennessee
1915 White Ave., Suite 107
Knoxville, TN 37916
(615) 971-1317

Texas

Cancer Information Service
UT M.D. Anderson Cancer Center
1515 Holcombe Blvd., #229
Houston, Texas 77030
(713) 792-3363

Utah

Cancer Information Service of Utah
University of Utah Health Science Center
50 N. Medical Dr.
Salt Lake City, UT 84132
(801) 581-5052

Washington

Cancer Information Service
Mailstop B-601-L
Fred Hutchinson Cancer Research Center
1124 Columbia St.
Seattle, WA 98104
(206) 467-4675

West Virginia

Cancer Information Service
Mary Babb Randolph Cancer Center
510 Medical Center Dr.
West Virginia University
Morgantown, WV 26506
(304) 293-2370

Wisconsin (and Iowa)

Cancer Information Service
1300 University Ave., 7C
Madison, WI 53706
(608) 262-0046

National CIS

Cancer Information Service
Biospherics, Inc.
12051 Indiana Creek Ct.
Beltsville, MD 20705
(301) 369-3900

Appendix C

CIS Call Record Form and Code Sheet

CIS CALL RECORD FORM

CIS Office [1][2] Case [3][4][5][6][7][8][9] Staff I.D. [10][11][12][13] Date MONTH [14][15] DAY [16][17] YEAR [18][19] ___1.Telephone ___2.Mail ___3.Walk in [20]

Type of Caller [21][22]

01-Patient, diagnosed by physician
02-Undiagnosed person with symptoms - has *not* been to a physician
03-Undiagnosed person with symptoms - *has* been to physician
04-Spouse, relative, friend of diagnosed patient
05-Spouse, relative, friend of a person with undiagnosed symptoms who has *not* been to a physician
06-Spouse, relative, friend of a person with undiagnosed symptoms who *has* been to a physician
07-General public
08-ACS representative/volunteer
09-Physician
10-Nurse
11-Social Worker
12-Other health professional/ organization
13-Educator
14-Clergy
15-Librarian
16-Media
17-Student/parent calling for student
18-Other non-health professionals
19-Not able to ascertain
20-Other CIS

Narrative description of inquiry and response

Subject of Inquiry [23][24] [25][26] [27][28] [29][30] [31][32]

Primary Cancer Site/Type [33][34] [35][36] [37][38]

Medical Disclaimer (lay public only): [39]
"I have given you our most accurate and up-to-date information. However, you should keep in mind that I am not a medical doctor. If you have requested this information because of your own medical condition or for someone you know, the information I have given you should be discussed with your physician. Only a physician, who has a complete medical history of a person can determine what is advisable in that particular case."

Medical Disclaimer given ______ 1. Yes ______ 2. No

Known high risk (do not ask) [40][41]

01-Smoking/tobacco use
02-DES
03-Asbestos
04-Radiation treatments for non-malignant conditions of head or neck
05-Family history of breast cancer
06-Familial polyposis
07- ____________________
08- ____________________
09-Not discussed /not appliciable

Did the inquiry relate to a metastatic cancer? ______ 1. Yes ______ 2. No or unknown [42]

CALLER IDENTIFICATION

Phone Number: (   ) ____________________

Case Number: ____________________

Name: ____________________

Address: ____________________

____
City/State/Zip

Behavioral suggestions/referrals (circle up to 5)

01-Talk to or visit a physician (has no personal physician)
02-Talk to or visit a physician (has a personal physician)
03-Seek a second opinion
04-Learn/practice self-detection technique
05-Attempt to stop/reduce smoking
06-Reduce the exposure to other health hazards
07-Share cancer information obtained with other person(s)
08-Tell person to call the CIS
09-Read literature

Contact Other Agency or Service
10-ACS
11-Hospital/Clinic
12-NCI or NCI-designated comprehensive or specialized cancer center or cooperative group
13-County/local medical association/physician referral
14-Counseling/support group
15-Hospice
16-Other community agency or service
17-No behavioral suggestion appropriate
18-Other ______________
20-Use PDQ

Sex of Caller _____ 1. Male _____ 2. Female

We are always trying to improve our service. Would you mind helping us by answering a few short questions?

Have you ever used our service before? _____ 1. Yes _____ 2. No _____ 3. Did not ask

How did you first find out about the CIS? (circle 1)

01-Relative
02-Friend/neighbor/co-worker
03-Physician
04-ACS
05-Other health professional/agency
06-Other CIS Office/backup WATS
07-TV
08-Radio
09-Newspaper
10-Newsletter/magazine
11-Brochure/pamphlet/book
12-Telephone book
13-Directory assistance/"800" information
14-CIS Parent Organization
15-Poster
16-Other ______________
17-Caller gave no information
18-Did not ask
19-Previous user
20-TV, Specific ______________
21-TV, Specific ______________
30-Radio, Specific ______________
31-Radio, Specific ______________
40-Newspaper, Specific ______________
41-Newspaper, Specific ______________
50-Newsletter, Magazine, Specific ______________
51-Newsletter, Magazine, Specific ______________
52-Other, Specific ______________
53-Other, Specific ______________

Age of Caller (Lay public only)
(1) 19 or less
(2) 20-29
(3) 30-39
(4) 40-49
(5) 50-59
(6) 60 or over
(7) No information given
(8) Did not ask
(9) Previous user

Education of Caller (Lay public only)
1- Grade school
2- Some High School
3- High School Graduate
4- Some College
5- College Graduate
6- Post-graduate training
7- No information given
8- Did not ask
9- Previous user

Ethnic Background of Caller (Lay public only)
1- White, not of Hispanic origin
2- Black, not of Hispanic origin
3- Asian or Pacific Islander
4- Hispanic
5- American Indian or Alaska native
7- No information given
8- Did not ask
9- Previous user

Location of Caller/State ______________

Location of Caller/County or Zip Code ______________ 62 63 64

Thank you for helping us. Please call again if you have any further questions on cancer.

Time to Handle Inquiry (on the phone) (1) None (2) 1-5 Minutes (3) 6-15 Minutes (4) 16-25 Minutes (5) More than 25 Minutes

Time to Handle Inquiry (Follow-up/Research) (1) None (2) 1-5 Minutes (3) 6-15 Minutes (4) 16-25 Minutes (5) More than 25 Minutes

Follow-up (circle up to 5)
1- None
2- Call back
3- Letter
4- User survey
5- Send publications
6- Other ______________
7- PDQ mailed

69 70 71 72

Primary Language Used During Call 1- English 2- Spanish 3- Other ______________

75 76 77 78

PDQ Resources Used 1-NCI Hard Copy of PDQ 2-Online PDQ Search 3-NCI Hard Copy and PDQ Search
File Used
01-Protocols
02-Cancer Information
03-Physicians
04-Organizations
05-Protocols and Cancer Information
06-Protocols and Physicians
07-Protocols and Organizations
08-Cancer Information and Physicians
09-Cancer Information and Organizations
10-Physicians and Organizations
11-Protocols, Cancer Information and Physicians
12-Protocols, Cancer Information and Organizations
13-Cancer Information, Physicians and Organizations
14-Physicians, Organizations and Protocols
15-Protocols, Cancer Information, Physicians and Organizations

Revis

CIS CALL RECORD FORM CODES

SUBJECT OF INQUIRY

01-CIS
02-CIS parent organization
03-NCI
04-ACS and other cancer-concerned organizations
05-Physician referral/second opinion
06-Hospitals/clinics/screening programs
07-Financial aid
08-Coping/counseling
09-Hospice
10-Equipment/supplies
11-Transportation
12-Home care/visiting nurse
13-Doctor/patient relationship
14-Statistics
15-Donations
16-Diet and Nutrition (Prevention)
17-Consultation between professionals
18-Site information, general or other
19-Diet and Nutrition (Patient)
20-Other primary prevention
21-Screening - Pap Smear
22-Screening - Breast Self Exam
23-Screening - Guaiac Test
24-Screening - Other
25-Symptoms
26-Diagnosis/diagnostic tests

Risk Factors
27-Risk factors, general
28-DES
29-Other specific drugs, food additives
30-Radiation
31-Heredity
32-Smoking/tobacco use
33-Asbestos
34-Other occupational risks
35-Lifestyle
36-Sun exposure
37-Other causes/risk factors

Treatment
38-Treatment, general
39-Surgery
40-Radiotherapy
41-Chemotherapy
42-Hormonal therapy
43-Biological Response Modifiers
44-Clinical trials
45-Other research
46-Unproven methods/quackery
47-Side effects/complication

48-Metastasis
49-Pain control
50-Physical and occupational rehabilitation
51-Prognosis

52-Publications/educational materials (bulk orders)
53-Publications/educational materials (5 or less)

54-Non-cancer call
55-Other ________________
56-General Cancer
57-PDQ
60-79-(PCCL categories)

PRIMARY CANCER SITE/TYPE

01-Breast
02-Bone
03-Connective and other soft tissue
04-Eye
05-Thyroid gland
06-Kaposi's Sarcoma

Digestive System
10-Mouth
11-Esophagus
12-Stomach
13-Small intestine
14-Colon
15-Rectum
16-Liver
17-Pancreas
18-Other or unspecified or digestive system, general

Respiratory System
30-Nasal cavity
31-Larynx
32-Lung/Trachea/Bronchus
33-Other or unspecified or respiratory system, general
34-Other or unspecified or head and neck, general

Genital System
40-Cervix
41-Uterus
42-Ovary, fallopian tubes
43-Other or unspecified or female genital, general
44-Prostate
45-Testes
46-Other or unspecified or male genital, general

Urinary System
50-Bladder
51-Kidney
52-Wilm's Tumor
53-Other or unspecified or urinary system, general

Lymphatic and Circulatory System
60-Hodgkin's Disease
61-Non-Hodgkin's Lymphoma
62-Multiple Myeloma
63-Leukemia
64-Heart
65-Other or unspecified or general, lymphatic or circulatory system

Central Nervous System
70-Brain
71-Spinal cord
72-Other or unspecified or CNS, general

Skin
80-Melanoma of skin
81-Non-melanoma skin cancer
82-Other or unspecified or skin cancer, general

90-Primary Site unknown
91-Other
92-AIDS
99-No specific site mentioned

LOCATION OF CALLER/STATE

01-Alabama
02-Alaska
03-Arizona
04-Arkansas
05-California
06-Colorado
07-Connecticut
08-Delaware
09-District of Columbia
10-Florida
11-Georgia
12-Hawaii
13-Idaho
14-Illinois
15-Indiana
16-Iowa
17-Kansas
18-Kentucky
19-Louisiana
20-Maine
21-Maryland
22-Massachusetts
23-Michigan
24-Minnesota
25-Mississippi
26-Missouri
27-Montana
28-Nebraska
29-Nevada
30-New Hampshire
31-New Jersey
32-New Mexico
33-New York City
34-New York State
35-North Carolina
36-North Dakota
37-Ohio
38-Oklahoma
39-Oregon
40-Pennsylvania
41-Rhode Island
42-South Carolina
43-South Dakota
44-Tennessee
45-Texas
46-Utah
47-Vermont
48-Virginia
49-Washington
50-West Virginia
51-Wisconsin
52-Wyoming
53-Puerto Rico
54-Canada
55-Mexico
56-Other Foreign Countries

Revised 2/86

Appendix D

CIS User Survey

A Survey of Cancer Information Service Callers

You recently called the Cancer Information Service (CIS). We hope you were able to obtain the information you needed. We would appreciate your assistance in improving our service by filling out this questionnaire. Although you are not required to do so, it would be a great help to us if you answered all the questions in this form. Your answers will be kept strictly confidential.

Please return the completed questionnaire in the enclosed postage-paid envelope. If the Cancer Information Service can be of help to you in the future, please feel free to contact us. Thank you for your help.

S ____________

The following questions refer to the call you made recently to the Cancer Information Service (CIS). Please check the appropriate answers.

	YES	NO
1. When you first decided to call the CIS, did you:		
a. Have difficulty obtaining the CIS telephone number?	____	____
b. Reach the wrong number?	____	____
c. Get a busy signal?	____	____
d. Have to call back because no one answered the phone?	____	____
2. When you first spoke with someone at the CIS:		
a. At any time during your conversation, did the person put you on hold for an unreasonable length of time?	____	____
b. Were you asked to call back because a counselor was not immediately available?	____	____

	YES	NO
c. Were you told that someone would call you back because a counselor was not immediately available?	____	____
(1) If yes, did a counselor call you back within the next working day?	____	____
d. Was the person you spoke with courteous?	____	____
e. Was the person you spoke with knowledgeable?	____	____
f. Was the person you spoke with friendly and sympathetic?	____	____
3. Please answer the questions below regarding your call to CIS:		
a. Was the information helpful?	____	____
b. Was the information clear and easy to understand?	____	____
c. Was most of the information new to you?	____	____
d. If some of the information you received from CIS was not new to you, please answer questions 1 and 2 below.		
1. Was the information you received from CIS in agreement with what you already knew before you called CIS?	____	____
2. Was the CIS information more informative than what you had obtained from other sources?	____	____
4. If you have other questions about cancer, will you call the CIS again?	____	____
5. Have you recommended the CIS to others since you used it?	____	____
6. Was your <u>most important question</u> answered by the CIS?	____	____

a. What was your most important question?

____

____

7. Which of the following statements <u>best</u> describes the reason you called the CIS? (Check <u>all</u> that apply)

____ a. I needed an explanation of something I heard (or read) from another source.

____ b. I wanted to know if the information I obtained from another source was correct.

____ c. I wanted to obtain a pamphlet which was advertised on TV or radio.

____ d. I wanted to obtain a pamphlet which was advertised in a magazine or newspaper.

____ e. I wanted to obtain information I could not find elsewhere.

_____ f. I wanted a referral to a physician, agency or service.

_____ g. I needed someone to talk to.

_____ h. Other, please specify ____________________

8. Which of the following did you like <u>most</u> about the CIS? (Check <u>all</u> that apply)

_____ a. The prompt response when I called.

_____ b. The counselor was courteous and sympathetic.

_____ c. The counselor helped me with my problem.

_____ d. The information was useful.

_____ e. The information was free of charge.

_____ f. The information was clear and understandable.

_____ g. Other, please specify ____________________

9. Which of the following did you like least about the CIS? (Check <u>all</u> that apply)

_____ a. The telephone number was hard to find.

_____ b. The telephone lines were often busy.

_____ c. The counselor was not immediately available.

_____ d. The counselor was not courteous or sympathetic.

_____ e. I was given outdated information.

_____ f. The information was not explained well.

_____ g. Other, please specify ____________________

_____ h. Nothing was unsatisfactory.

10. If printed materials (other than this survey) were sent to you, such as pamphlets or brochures, what did you do with them? (Check <u>all</u> that apply)

_____ (1) I never received the materials.

_____ (2) I read all the materials sent to me.

_____ (3) I read part of the materials sent to me.

_____ (4) I have not yet read them.

_____ (5) I gave them to others to read.

_____ (6) Other, please specify ____________________

_____ (7) No printed materials were sent to me.

11. How would you rate your overall satisfaction with the Cancer Information Service? Would you say that you are: (Check only <u>one</u>)

_____ a. Very satisfied

_____ b. Somewhat satisfied

_____ c. Neither satisfied nor dissatisfied

_____ d. Somewhat dissatisfied

_____ e. Very dissatisfied

12. Some callers to the CIS are given suggestions for actions to take following their call. Since calling the CIS, what action, or actions, have you taken regarding the question(s) you asked? (Check all that apply.)

____ a. I went to, or made an appointment with, my regular physician.

____ b. I sought a second opinion from another physician.

____ c. I went to or made an appointment with the physician, clinic, or hospital to which I was referred by the CIS.

____ d. I contacted the community agency or service to which I was referred.

____ e. I read the printed materials that were mailed to me.

____ f. I learned and/or practiced the cancer self-detection technique I was told about, such as breast self-examination.

____ g. I attempted to stop or reduce smoking.

____ h. I attempted to reduce my exposure to environmental health hazards. For example, I started wearing protective equipment at work or reduced time spent in the sun, etc.

____ i. I changed my eating habits.

____ j. I sought more information about my question.

____ k. I shared the information I received from CIS with at least one other person. Of the people you shared the information with, how many were:

a. male ________

b. female ________

____ l. I took no action. (If you took no action, please skip from here to Question 15.)

____ m. Other, please specify ________________

13. Sometimes peoples' actions are influenced by many individuals or sources. Did any of the following influence any of the actions which you checked in Question 12? (Check all that apply)

____ a. Relatives and/or friends

____ b. My physician

____ c. Other health professionals, such as a nurse or pharmacist

____ d. Other cancer organizations, such as the American Cancer Society

____ e. TV/Radio

____ f. Newspapers/Magazines

____ g. Scientific or professional magazines or journals

____ h. Other, please specify ________________

____ i. None of these individuals or sources influenced my course of action

14. Keeping in mind all of the individuals or sources that influenced you, how important was your contact with the CIS in your

decision to take the action you specified in Question 12? (Check only one)

____ a. Very important

____ b. Somewhat important

____ c. Not very important

____ d. Not important at all

	YES	NO
15. When you called the CIS, were you referred to a person or agency that you had not contacted before? If no, please skip from here to Question 17.	____	____
16. Have you contacted that person or agency?	____	____
a. If yes, was the person or agency able to provide the service that the CIS indicated they could?	____	____

17. To help us decide if our hours of service are convenient,

a. When would you prefer to call the CIS? (Check all that apply)

____ (1) 8:00 A.M. to Noon, Monday–Friday

____ (2) 12:01 P.M. to 5:00 P.M., Monday–Friday

____ (3) 5:01 P.M. to Midnight, Monday–Friday

____ (4) Weekends

b. Are you: (Check all that apply)

____ (1) Employed full-time

____ (2) Not employed

____ (3) Employed part-time

____ (4) Retired

____ (5) A homemaker

____ (6) A student

If you wish to comment further on the Cancer Information Service, please use the space below.

____

____

____

____

____

____

____

____

____

____

THANK YOU FOR YOUR PARTICIPATION

Appendix E

Selected CIS Data Tables

Family/friends are combined with their respective caller groups in these tables, unlike the chapter text where they are usually separated for discussion purposes.

Subject of Inquiry
Cancer Information Service, 1983–86

Subject of inquiry	All symptomatic persons and family/ friends	General public	Cancer patients and family/ friends
Local organizations and services; physician referral	24.3	7.7	37.0
Diet and nutrition	.7	10.7	2.7
General cancer information	17.5	15.0	27.8
Prevention	1.2	31.0	1.8
Screening	5.0	2.4	.6
Symptoms	50.1	3.4	2.7
Diagnotic tests	18.1	1.5	3.9
Risk factors	7.3	43.7	4.3
Treatment	8.3	2.0	40.2
Continuing care	3.5	.6	17.0

Cancer Sites Most Frequently Asked About

Cancer Information Service, 1983–86

Site/type	All symptomatic persons and family/ friends	General public	Cancer patients and family/ friends
Breast	49.0	37.7	29.6
Lung/trachea/bronchus	7.1	14.9	16.5
Colon/rectum	15.3	19.6	12.7
Leukemia	2.4	6.4	6.4
Prostate	2.8	2.8	7.2
Melanoma of skin	4.0	3.1	5.5
Non-Hodgkin's lymphoma	1.4	1.3	6.1
Cervix	6.0	5.9	3.0
Other skin	7.7	7.7	1.2
Hodgkin's disease	1.7	1.5	3.5
Brain	1.4	1.5	3.9
Uterus	2.8	2.6	2.6
Pancreas	1.1	1.0	3.6

How Different User Groups First Learned of the CIS

Cancer Information Service, 1983–86

How did you first find out about the CIS?	All symptomatic persons and family/ friends	General public	Cancer patients and family/ friends
Relative	2.7	1.4	4.2
Friend/neighbor/co-worker	7.1	3.9	9.4
Physician	.6	.4	1.7
ACS	8.3	3.9	11.1
Other health professional/agency	3.2	1.8	5.1
Other CIS Office/backup WATS	4.5	1.1	4.6
TV	19.8	52.5	11.3
Radio	2.0	7.9	1.3
Newspaper	5.4	6.9	5.5
Newsletter/magazine	7.1	3.2	5.4
Brochure/pamphlet/book	8.7	3.4	12.4
Telephone book	19.8	6.8	14.9
Directory assistance/"800" information	5.0	1.6	4.7
CIS parent organization	3.0	1.5	5.2
Poster	.2	.2	.1
Other	2.5	3.4	2.7

Behavioral Suggestions for Different CIS User Groups

Cancer Information Service, 1983–86

Behavioral suggestion	All symptomatic persons and family/friends	General public	Cancer patients and family/friends
Talk to or visit a physician (has no personal physician)	8.9	.7	1.0
Talk to or visit a physician (has a personal physician)	54.7	5.6	31.9
Seek a second opinion	13.6	.8	9.8
Learn/practice self-detection techniques	1.8	1.9	.4
Attempt to stop/reduce smoking	1.6	23.9	.5
Reduce the exposure to other health hazards	.6	2.5	.3
Share cancer information obtained with other person(s)	5.3	8.6	11.9
Tell person to call the CIS	12.0	7.2	14.1
Read literature	26.6	63.2	37.2
Contact other agency or service			
ACS	2.0	5.1	8.8
Hospital/clinic	8.5	1.9	6.5
NCI or NCI-designated comprehensive or specialized cancer center or cooperative group	9.1	2.3	23.0
County/local medical association	7.7	.8	4.5
Counseling/support group	.7	1.0	4.6
Hospice	.0	.1	1.8
Other community agency or service	3.3	8.4	7.9
Other	1.1	2.4	2.6

Appendix F

List of NCI Cancer Communications Research Grantees

Illinois Cancer Council, Chicago, Illinois

"Information Seeking Behavior of Cancer Patients"
Clara Manfredi, Ph.D.
Illinois Cancer Council
36 South Wabash Ave., Suite 700
Chicago, IL 60603
(312)346-9813

Roswell Park Memorial Institute, Buffalo, New York

"Effectiveness of Targeted Anti-smoking Communications"
K. Michael Cummings, Ph.D.
Department of Cancer Control and Epidemiology
Roswell Park Memorial Institute
666 Elm St.
Buffalo, NY 14263
(716)845-8456

Fred Hutchinson Cancer Research Center, Seattle, Washington

"Test of a Telephone Intervention for Blue Collar Smokers"
Maureen M. Henderson, M.D.
Program Head, Cancer Prevention Research Program
Fred Hutchinson Cancer Research Center
1124 Columbia St.
Seattle, WA 98104
(206) 467-4678

University of California, Los Angeles, California

"Promotion of Mammography Screening Using the CIS"
Alfred C. Marcus, Ph.D.
Jonsson Comprehensive Cancer Center at UCLA
1100 Glendon Ave., Suite 711
Los Angeles, CA 90024
(213)206-0278

University of Maryland, College Park, Maryland

"Narrowing the Cancer Knowledge Gap Among Blacks"
Vicki Freimuth, Ph.D., Associate Professor
1136 Tawes Fine Arts
University of Maryland
College Park, MD 20742
(301)454-5813

References

Abrams, R.D. (1966). The patient with cancer—his changing pattern of communication. *New England Journal of Medicine*, 274(6), 317–322.

Adams, M., and Kerner, J. (1982). Evaluation of promotional strategies to solve the problem of underutilization of a breast examination center in a New York City black community. In C. Mettlin and G.P. Murphy (eds.), *Issues in Cancer Screening and Communications*. New York: Alan R. Liss, Inc.

Altman, D. (1984/1985). Evaluation of the cancer information service: Implications for health behavior and health services research (doctoral dissertation, University of California at Irvine, 1984/1985). *Dissertation Abstracts International*, 45-09, 2884-B.

American Cancer Society. (1985). *Cancer in the Economically Disadvantaged*. New York: American Cancer Society.

———. (1987). *1987 Cancer Facts and Figures*. New York: American Cancer Society.

Antonovsky, A., and Hartman, H. (1974). Delay in the detection of cancer: A review of the literature. *Health Education Monographs*, 2(2), 98–128.

Atkin, C.K. (1973). Instrumental utilities and information seeking. In P. Clarke (ed.), *New Models for Mass Communication Research* (pp. 205–242). Beverly Hills, California: Sage Publications.

———. (1979). Research evidence on mass mediated health communications campaigns. In D. Nimmo (ed.), *Communication Yearbook 3* (pp. 655–668). New Brunswick, New Jersey: Transaction Books.

Baquet, C., and Ringen, K. (1986). Cancer control in blacks: Epidemiology and NCI program plans. In L.E. Mortenson, P.F. Engstrom and P.N. Anderson (eds.), *Advances in Cancer Control: Health Care Financing and Research* (pp. 215–227). New York: Alan R. Liss, Inc.

Barbarin, O.A., and Chesler, M.A. (1984). Relationships with the medical staff and aspects of satisfaction with care expressed by parents of children with cancer. *Journal of Community Health*, 9(4), 302–313.

Bartlett, M.H., Johnson, A., and Meyer, T.C. (1973). Dial-access library-patient information service. *New England Journal of Medicine*, 228(19), 994–997.

Bergner, L., and Yerby, A.S. (1968). Low income and barriers to use of health services. *New England Journal of Medicine*, 278(10), 541–546.

Bertakis, K.D. (1977). The communication of information from physicians to patient: A method for increasing patient retention and satisfaction. *Journal of Family Practice*, 5(2), 217–222.

Betteman, J.R. (1979). *An Information Processing Theory of Consumer Choice*. Reading, Massachusetts: Addison-Wesley.

Birch, D.L. (1981). Who creates jobs? *The Public Interest*, 65, 3–14.

Block, C.E. (1972). Prepurchase search behavior of low-income households. *Journal of Retailing*, 48(1), 3–15.

Boreham, P., and Gibson, D. (1978). The informative process in private medical consultations: A preliminary investigation. *Social Science and Medicine*, 12, 409–416.

Brown, J.M., Helling, D.K., Burns, E.A., Burmeister, L.F., and Rakel, R.E. (1982). Patient care telephone calls received in family practice offices. *Journal of Family Practice*, 14(3), 527–532.

Butler, M., and Paisley, W. (1976). The potential of mass communication and interpersonal communication for cancer control. In J.W. Cullen, B.H. Fox, and R.N. Isom (eds.), *Cancer: The Behavioral Dimensions* (pp. 205–229). New York: Raven Press.

———. (1977). Communicating cancer control to the public. *Health Education Monograph*, 5(1), 5–24.

Carothers, J.E., and Inslee, L.J. (1974). Level of empathic understanding offered by volunteer telephone services. *Journal of Counseling Psychology*, 21, 274–276.

Cassileth, B.R., Zupkis, R.V., Sutton-Smith, K., and March, V. (1980). Information and participation preferences among cancer patients. *Annals of Internal Medicine*, 92(6), 832–836.

Catanzaro, R.J., and Green, W.G. (1970). Wats telephone therapy: New follow-up techniques for alcoholics. *American Journal of Psychiatry*, 126, 1024–1027.

Cherry, C. (1977). The telephone system: Creator of mobility and social change. In I. Pool (ed.), *The Social Impact of the Telephone* (pp. 112–126). Cambridge, Massachusetts: MIT Press.

Childers, T., and Post, J.A. (1975). *The Information Poor in America*. Metuchen, New Jersey: Scarecrow Press.

Comaroff, T., and Maguire, P. (1981). Ambiguity and the search for meaning: Childhood leukaemia in the modern clinical context. *Social Science and Medicine*, 15B, 115–123.

Cooke, T.D., Appleton, H., Conner, R.F., Shaffer, A., Tamkin, G., and Weber, S.J. (1975). *"Sesame Street" Revisited*. New York: Russell Sage Foundation.

Dervin, B. (1976). Strategies for dealing with human information needs: Information or communication? *Journal of Broadcasting*, 20, (3)324–333.

——— (1980). Communication gaps and inequities: Moving toward a reconceptualization. In B. Dervin and M.J. Voigt (Eds.), *Progress in Communication Sciences* (Vol. 2, pp. 73–112). Norwood, New Jersey: Ablex.

Dervin, B., Zweizig, D., Hall, E.P., Kwaii, C., and Lalley R. (1977). The Development of strategies for dealing with the information needs of urban residents: Phase II-Information practitioner study. (Final report on Project No. 475 AH 50014 to Office of Libraries and Learning Resources, Office of Education, U.S. Department of Health, Education, and Welfare.) (ED 136791).

DeVita, V.T., Jr. (1986). Responsible reporting of an emotional issue. *SIPI-scope*, Summer. pp. 8–9.

Dunwoody, S. (1980). The science writing inner club: A communication link between science and the lay public. *Science, Technology and Human Values*, 5(30), 14–22.

Eakin, D., Jackson, S.J., and Hannigan, G.G. (1980). Consumer health information: Libraries as partners. *Bulletin of the Medical Library Association*, 68(2), 220–229.

Eardley, A. (1974). Triggers to action: A study of what makes women seek advice for breast conditions. *International Journal of Health Education*, 17, 256–265.

Eckert, D. (1983). A methodology for cancer control utilizing cancer information service data. In C. Mettlin and G.P. Murphy (eds.), *Progress in Cancer Control IV: Research in the Cancer Center* (pp. 161–170). New York: Alan R. Liss, Inc.

Egbert, L.D., Battit, G.E., Welch, C.E., and Bartlett, M.K. (1964). Reduction of postoperative pain by encouragement and instruction of patients. *New England Journal of Medicine*, 270(16), 825–827.

Ellis, D.A., Hopkin, J., Leitch, A.G., and Crofton, J. (1979). Doctors' Orders: Controlled trial of supplementary written information for patients. *British Medical Journal*, 1, 456.

Ettema, J.S. (1984). Three phases in the creation of information inequities: An empirical assessment of a prototype videotext system. *Journal of Broadcasting*, 28(4), 389–395.

Ettema, J.S., Brown, J.W., and Luepker, R.V. (1983). Knowledge gap effects in a health information campaign. *Public Opinion Quarterly*, 47, 516–527.

Ettema, J.S., and Kline, F.G. (1977). Deficits, differences, and ceilings: Contingent conditions for understanding the knowledge gap. *Communication-Research*, 4(2), 179–202.

Evans, S.H., and Clarke, P. (1983). When cancer patients fail to get well: Flaws in health communication. In R.N. Bostrom (ed.), *Communication Yearbook* 7, (pp. 225–248). Beverly Hills, California: Sage Publications, Inc.

FDC Reports, Inc. (1988, February 3). Breakthrough cancer treatments have not been used in large numbers. *The Blue Sheet*, 31(5), 2.

Ferguson, J.A. (1983). *Evaluating the Cancer Communications Network National Data Collecting Instrument*. Unpublished master's thesis, University of Alabama School of Public Health, Birmingham, Alabama.

Flay, B. (1986). Mass media and smoking cessation. Paper presented to the International Communication Association, Montreal, May.

Flay, B.R., DiTecco, D., and Schlegel, R.P. (1980). Mass media in health promotion: An analysis using an extended information-processing model. *Health Education Quarterly*, 7(2), 127–147.

Fowler, G.D., and Wackerbarth, M.E. (1980). Audio teleconferencing versus face-to-face conferencing: A synthesis of literature. *Western Journal of Speech Communication*, 44, 236–252.

Freimuth, V.S. (1979). Assessing the readability of health education messages. *Public Health Reports*, 94(6), 568–570.

Freimuth, V.S., Greenberg, R.H., DeWitt, J., and Romano, R.M. (1984). Covering cancer: Newspapers and the public interest. *Journal of Communication* 34(1), 62–73.

Freimuth, V.S., and Van Nevel, J.P. (1981). Reaching the public: The asbestos awareness campaign. *Journal of Communication*, 31(2), 155–167.

Gaziano, C. (1983). The knowledge gap: An analytical review of media effects. *Communication Research*, 10(4), 447–486.

Genova, B.K.L., and Greenberg, B.S. (1979). Interests in news and the knowledge gap. *Public Opinion Quarterly*, 43(1), 79–91.

Gerbner, G., Gross, L., Morgan, M., and Signorielli, N. (1981). Health and medicine on television. *New England Journal of Medicine*, 305, 901–904.

Goldsen, R.K., Gerhardt, P.K., and Handy, V.H. (1963). Patient delay in seeking cancer treatment: Behavioral aspects. *Journal of Chronic Diseases*, 16, 427–436.

Goodman, E. (1985). Speaking of cancer. *The Washington Post*. July 20, A-19.

Gotay, C.C. (1984). The experience of cancer during early and advanced stages: The views of patients and their mates. *Social Science and Medicine*, 18(7), 605–613.

Green, L.W. (1976). Site- and symptom-related factors in secondary prevention of cancer. In J.W. Cullen, B.H. Fox, and R.N. Isom (eds.), *Cancer: The Behavioral Dimensions*. New York: Raven Press.

Greenberg, R. (1986). *1984 Content Analysis of Newspaper Coverage of Cancer*. Bethesda, Maryland: National Cancer Institute.

Hammond, S.L., Freimuth, V.S., and Morrison, W. (1987). The gatekeeping funnel: Tracking a major PSA campaign from distribution through gatekeepers to target audience. *Health Education Quarterly*, 14(2), 153–166.

Haug, M., and Lavin, B. (1983). *Consumerism in Medicine: Challenging Physician Authority*, Beverly Hills, California: Sage Publications.

Heagerty, M.C., Robertson, L., Kosa, J., and Alpert, J.J. (1968). Use of the telephone by low income families. *Journal of Pediatrics*, 73(5), 740–744.

Hulka, B.S., Cassel, J.C., Kupper, L.L., and Burdette, J.A. (1976). Communication, compliance, and concordance between physicians and patients with prescribed medications. *American Journal of Public Health*, 66, 847–853.

Janofsky, A.I. (1971). Affective self-disclosure in telephone versus face-to-face interviews. *Journal of Humanistic Psychology*, 11, 93–103.

Johnson, J.E. (1973). Effects of accurate expectations about sensations on the sensory and distress components of pain. *Journal of Personality and Social Psychology*, 27(2), 261–275.

Johnson, J.E., Fuller, S.S., Endress, M.P., and Rice, V.H. (1978). Altering patients' responses to surgery: An extension and replication. *Research in Nursing and Health*, 1(3), 111–121.

Johnson, J.E., and Leventhal, H. (1974). Effects of accurate expectations and behavioral instructions on reactions during a noxious medical examination. *Journal of Personality and Social Psychology*, 29(5), 710–718.

Johnson, J.E., and Rice, V.H. (1974). Sensory and distress components of pain: Implications for the study of clinical pain. *Nursing Research*, 23(3), 203–208.

Korsch, B.M., Gozzi, E.K., and Francis, V. (1968). Gaps in doctor-patient communication, 1. Doctor-patient interaction and patient satisfaction. *Pediatrics*, 42(5), 855–871.

Kozol, J. (1985). *Illiterate America*. New York: Anchor Press/Doubleday.

Kramer, R., Docter, D., Mckenna, R., Irwin, L., Hisserich, J., and Hammond, G. (1981). Implementation and evaluation of a cancer information service. *International Quarterly of Community Health Education*, 1(2), 153–168.

Krant, M.J., and Johnston, L. (1978). Family members' perceptions of communications in late stage cancer. *International Journal of Psychiatry in Medicine*, 8(2), 203–216.

Landis, D. (1985). Cancer dilemma tested marketers' ethics, good taste. *Adweek*, September 23, pp. 42–44.

Lee, J., Kline, F.G., Jacobs, D.R., Jr., and Hannan, P.J. (1985). Acquisition of health messages for different individual and family types in different communities. Paper presented at the annual meeting of ICA, May 1985, Honolulu.

Lenz, E.R. (1979). Newcomers' search for information about health services. In E. Bowens (Ed.), *Clinical Nursing Research: Its Strategies and Findings* (pp. 182–189). Indianapolis, Sigma Theta Tau.

Lenz, E.R. (1984). Information seeking: A component of client decisions and health behavior. *Advances in Nursing Science*, 6(3), 59–72.

Leventhal, H., Safer, M.A., and Panagis, D.M. (1983). The impact of communications on the self-regulation of health beliefs, decisions, and behavior. *Health Education Quarterly*, 10(1), 3–29.

Levy, A.S., and Stokes, R.C. (1987). Effects of health promotion advertising campaign on sales of ready-to-eat cereals. *Public Health Reports*, 102(4), 398–403.

Ley, P. (1972a). Primacy, rated importance and the recall of medical information. *Journal of Health and Social Behavior*, 13, 311–317.

——— (1972b). Comprehension, memory and the success of communications with the patient. *Journal of the Institute of Health Education*, 10, 23–29.

——— (1977). Psychological studies of doctor-patient communication. In S. Rachman (ed.), *Contributions to Medical Psychology* (Vol. 1). Oxford: Pergamon Press.

——— (1979). Psychological and behavioral factors in weight loss. In G.A. Bray (ed.), *Recent Advances in Obesity Research*, 2. Westport, CT: Technomic Publishing Co.

——— (1982). Giving information to patients. In J.R. Eiser (ed.), *Social Psychology and Behavioral Medicine* (pp. 339–374). London: John Wiley & Sons, Ltd.

——— (1983). Patients' understanding and recall in clinical communication failure. In D. Pendleton and J. Hasler (eds.), *Doctor-Patient Communication* (pp. 89–107). London: Academic Press.

Ley, P., Bradshaw, P.W., Eaves, D., and Walker, C.M. (1973). A method for increasing patients' recall of information presented by doctors. *Psychological Medicine*, 3, 217–220.

Lieberman Research, Inc. (1978). *A Basic Study of Public Attitudes Toward Cancer and Cancer Tests*. Washington, D.C.: American Cancer Society.

Lippert, B. (1984). Kellogg puts some moral fiber in its all-bran ads. *Adweek*, October 22, p. 40.

Long, M.C. (1978). Television: Help or hindrance to health education? *Health Education*, May/June, 9(3), 32–34.

Maccoby, N., and Solomon, D.S. (1981). Heart disease prevention: Community studies. In R.E. Rice and W.J. Paisley (eds.), *Public Communciation Campaigns*. (pp. 105–126). Beverly Hills, California: Sage Publications, Inc.

Macro Systems. (1986). *1984 Content Analysis of Newspaper Coverage of Cancer*. Report submitted to the Office of Cancer Communications, National-Cancer Institute.

Matza, M. (1985). Cancer sells. *Boston Phoenix*, April 2, pp. 1, 8–9.

McDonald, M.D. (1986). *The Emergence of the Personal Health Information System*. Communication Technologies in Health Promotion. Conference, June, Bethesda, Maryland.

McIntosh, J. (1974). Progress of communication, information-seeking and control associated with cancer: A selective review of the literature. *Social Science and Medicine*, 8, 167–187.

McKnight, J.L. (1985). Where can health communication be found? Paper presented to the International Communication Association Convention, May 1985, Honolulu.

McLain, C. (1985). Back on her own feet. *10th Anniversary Yearbook*. Lexington, Kentucky: McDowell Cancer Network, 8–9.

Media's muscleman. (1977). *Media Decisions*, September, 64–65, 132–134.

Mendelsohn, H. (1976). Mass communications and cancer control. In J.W. Cullen, B.H. Fox, and R.N. Isom (eds.), *Cancer: The Behavioral Dimension* (pp.197–204). Bethesda, Maryland: National Cancer Institute.

Messerli, M.L., Garamendi, C., and Romano, J. (1980). Breast cancer: Information as a technique of crisis intervention. *American Journal Orthopsychiatry*, 50, 728–731.

Mettlin, C., Mirand, E., Sciandra, R., and Walsh, D. (1980). Public use of cancer information service. *Public Education About Cancer, UICC Technical Report Series*, 55.

Miller, M.H. (1973). Seeking advice for cancer symptoms. *American Journal of Public Health*, 63(11), 955–961.

Miller, S.M., and Managan, C.E. (1983). Interacting effects of information and coping style in adapting to gynecologic stress: Should the doctor tell all? *Journal of Personality and Social Psychology*, 45(1), 223–236.

Mitchell, G.W., and Glicksman, A.S. (1977). Cancer patients: Knowledge and attitudes. *Cancer*, 40(1), 61–66.

Naisbitt, J. (1984). *Megatrends*. New York: Warner Books, Inc.

National Analysts. (1982). National survey of public knowledge, attitudes, practices related to cancer. Prepared for Porter, Novelli, and Associates and Office of Cancer Communications, National Cancer Institute.

National Center for Health Statistics. (1987). Advance report of final mortality statistics, 1985. *Monthly Vital Statistics Report*, 36(5), Supplement DHHS Publication No. PHS 87-1120.

National Cancer Institute. (1983). *Public Attitudes and Behaviors Regarding Cancer Risk and Prevention*. Report prepared for Office of Cancer Communications.

——— (1986a). *Cancer Control Objectives for the Nation: 1985–2000* (NIH Publication No. 86–2880). Bethesda, Maryland: National Cancer Institute.

——— (1986b). *Physicians' Data Query Patient Education*. Bethesda, Maryland: National Institutes of Health.

——— (1986c). *Cancer Prevention Awareness Survey Wave II* (NIH Publication No. 87–2907). Bethesda, Maryland: National Cancer Institute.

——— (1986d). *1985 Annual Cancer Statistics Review*. Bethesda, Maryland: National Institutes of Health.

Neiman, F. (1984). All-Bran ads may inspire health trend. *Advertising Age*, October, 6–7.

Niemi, J.A., and Anderson, D.V. (1971). *Television: A Viable Channel for Educating Adults in Culturally Different Poverty Groups?—A Literature Review* (Report No. AC 010111). Syracuse, New York: Syracuse University. (ERIC Clearinghouse on Adult Education No. ED 048550).

Northouse, P.G. (1986). Communication and cancer: Issues confronting patients, health professionals and family members. Paper presented at the meeting of the Communicating with Patients Conference, Tampa, Florida, February.

Okie, S. (1986). Art imitates life and death. *Washington Post*, February 5, HW 12.

Olien, C.N., Donohue, G.A., and Tichenor, P.J. (1978). Community structure and media use. *Journalism Quarterly*, 55, 445–455.

Olien, C.N., Tichenor, P.J., and Donohue, G.A. (1982). Structure, communication, and social power: Evolution of the knowledge gap hypothesis. Paper presented at Sommatie '82 Conference, Veldhoven, the Netherlands, March 26.

O'Reilly, C.A., III. (1982). Variations in decision makers' use of information sources: The impact of quality and accessibility of information. *Academy of Management Journal*, 25(4), 756–771.

Orr, E. (1986). Open communication as an effective stress management method for breast cancer patients. *Journal of Human Stress*, 12(4), 175–185.

Parker, E.B., et al. (1966). *Patterns of Adult Information Seeking*. Stanford University, Institute for Communication Research. ERIC ED010–294.

Pendleton, D. (1983). Doctor-patient communication: A review. In D. Pendleton, and J. Hasler (eds.), *Doctor-Patient Communication* (pp. 5–53). London: Academic Press.

Pope, C.R., Yoshioka, S.S., and Greenlick, M.R. (1971). Determinants of medical care utilization: The use of the telephone for reporting symptoms. *Journal of Health and Social Behavior*, 12, 155–162.

Pratt, L. (1956). How do patients learn about disease? *Social Problems*, 4, 29–40.

Public attitudes toward cancer and cancer tests. (1980). *CA—A Cancer Journal for Clinicians*, 30(2), 92–98.

Rainey, L.C. (1985). Effects of preparatory patient education for radiation oncology patients. *Cancer*, 56(5), 1056–1061.

Reid, A.A.L. (1977). Comparing telephone with face-to-face contact. In I. Pool (ed.), *The Social Impact of the Telephone* (pp. 386–414). Cambridge, Massachusetts: MIT Press.

Rhetaugh, G.D., Anderson, B.J., and Leonard, R.C. (1965). The importance of the expressive function in preoperative preparation. In Skipper, J.K. and Leonard R.C. (eds.), *Social Interaction and Patient Care* (pp. 16–29). Philadelphia: J.B. Lippincott Company.

Richburg, K.B. (1985). Reports on cancer treatment cause a flood of inquiries. *Washington Post*, December 6, A3.

Robinson, J.P., and Levy, M.R. (1986). *The Main Source: Learning From Television News*. Beverly Hills, California: Sage Publications.

Rogers, E.M. (1983). *Diffusion of Innovations* (3rd ed.). New York: The Free Press.

Rogers, E.M., and Kincaid, D.L. (1981). *Communication Networks: Toward a New Paradigm for Research*. New York: The Free Press.

Rosenbaum, A., and Calhoun, J.F. (1977). The use of the telephone hotline in crisis intervention: A review. *Journal of Community Psychology*, 5(4), 325–339.

Rouse, W.B., and Rouse, S.H. (1984). Human information seeking and design of information systems. *Information Processing and Management*, 20(1–2), 129–138.

Sackett, D.L., Haynes, R.B., Gibson, E.S., Hackett, B.C., Taylor, D.W., Roberts, R.S., and Johnson, A.L. (1975). Randomized clinical trials of strategies for improving medication compliance in primary hypertension. *Lancet*, 1, 1205–1207.

Sandman, P.M. (1976). Medicine and mass communications: An agenda for physicians. *Annals of Internal Medicine*, 85(3), 378–383.

Schain, W.S. (1980). Patients' rights in decision making: The case for personalism versus paternalism in health care. *Cancer*, 46(4), 1035–1041.

Sciandra, R. and Stein, J. (1983). Applying marketing techniques to promotion of the cancer information service. In C. Mettlin and G.P. Murphy (eds.), *Progress In Cancer Control IV: Research in the Cancer Center* (pp. 153–160). New York: Alan R. Liss, Inc.

Schottenfeld, D., and Fraumeni, J.F. (1982). *Cancer Epidemiology and Prevention*. Philadelphia: W.B. Saunders.

Scully, T, and Scully, C. (1988). *Playing God: The New World of Medical Choices*. New York: Simon & Schuster.

Singer, B.D. (1981). *Social Functions of the Telephone*. Palo Alto, California: R & E Research Associates.

Skipper, J.K., and Leonard, R.C. (1968). Children, stress, and hospitalization: A field experiment. *Journal of Health and Social Behavior*, 9, 275–287.

Slaughter, E.P., Napolitano, C.S., and Freimuth, V.S. (1985). The Influence of Social Interaction on the Diffusion of Health Information. Paper presented at the meeting of the Health Communication Summer Conference, Chicago, Illinois.

Smith, F.A., Trivax, G., Zuehlke, D.A., Lowinger, P., and Nghiem, T.L. (1972). Health information during a week of television. *New England Journal of Medicine*, 286(10), 516–520.

Sontag, S. (1978). *Illness as Metaphor*. New York: Farrar, Straus & Giroux.

Staub, E., and Kellet, O.S. (1972). Increasing pain tolerance by information about aversive stimuli. *Journal of Personality and Social Psychology*, 21(2), 198–203.

Stein, J.A. and Kean, T.J. (1982). Quality assessment of the cancer information service: Evolution of a test call system. In *Issues in Cancer Screening and Communications* (pp. 469–483). New York: Alan R. Liss, Inc.

Stojanovic, E.J. (1972). The dissemination of information about medicare to low-income rural residents. *Rural Sociology*, 37, 253–260.

Stone, A.J., and Siegel, J.M. (1986). Correlates of accurate knowledge of cancer. *Health Education Quarterly*, 13(1), 39–50.

Stone, G.C. (1979). Patient compliance and the role of the expert. *Journal of Social Issues*, 35(1), 34–56.

Suchman, E.A. (1965). Social patterns of illness and medical care. *Journal of Health and Human Behavior*, 6, 2–16.

Tichenor, P.J., Donohue, G.A., and Olien, G.N. (1970). Mass media flow and differential growth in knowledge. *Public Opinion Quarterly*, 34(2), 158–170.

——— (1980). Conflict and the knowledge gap. In P.J. Tichenor (ed.), *Community Conflict and the Press*, (pp. 175–203). Beverly Hills, California: Sage Publications.

Toffler, A. (1970). *Future Shock*. New York: Random House.

Tuckett, D.A., Boulton, M., and Olson, C. (1985). A new approach to the measurement of patients understanding of what they are told in medical consultations. *Journal of Health and Social Behavior*, 26(1), 27–38.

Turow, J., and Coe, L. (1985). Curing television's ills: The portrayal of health care. *Journal of Communication*, 35(4), 36–51.

U.S. Bureau of the Census (1983). *1980 Census of Population and Housing*. Washington, D.C.: U.S. Government Printing Office.

U.S. Bureau of the Census. (1987). Current population reports, 1984. Series P60, No. 157, Table 16.

U.S. Department of Health, Education & Welfare. (1979). *Healthy People: The Surgeon General's Report on Health Promotion and Disease Prevention* (DHEW (PHS) Publication No. 79–55071). Washington, D.C.: U.S. Government Printing Office.

Vickery, D.M. and Fries, J.F. (1976). *Take Care of Yourself: A Consumer's Guide to Medical Care*. Reading, Massachusetts: Addison-Wesley.

Waitzkin, H. (1985). Information giving in medical care. *Journal of Health and Social Behavior*, 26, 81–101.

Waitzkin, H., and Stoeckle, J.D. (1972). The communication of information about illness. *Advances in Psychosomatic Medicine*, 8, 180–215.

Wark, V. (1982). A look at the work of the telephone counseling center. *Personnel and Guidance Journal*, 61, 110–112.

Weingarten, M.A. (1982). Telephone consultations with patients: A briefstudy and review of the literature. *Journal of the Royal College of General Practitioners*, 32, 766–770.

Whelan, E.M., Sheridan, J.J., Meister, K.A., and Mosher, B.A. (1981). Analysis of coverage of tobacco hazard in women's magazines. *Journal of Public Health Policy*, 2(1), 28–35.

Wilkinson, G.S., Mirand, E.A., and Graham, S. (1985). *An Evaluation of a Cancer Information Telephone Facility*. New York: Praeger.

Wolinsky, H. (1985). Using cancer to sell cereal: Breakthrough or bad news? *American College of Physicians Observer*, September, 4–5.

Wright, K., and Dyck, S. (1984). Expressed concerns of adult cancer patients' family members. *Cancer Nursing*, 7(5), 371–374.

Yarrow, A.L. (1987). The revolution wrought by toll-free calls. *New York Times*, February 12, C1.

Index